THE HEALTH ANSWER BOOK:

The Complete Guide to Symptoms, Causes, and Natural Cures for Hundreds of Health Problems

By the Editors of FC&A

FC&A
103 Clover Green
Peachtree City, GA 30269
Produced by the staff of FC&A

Second printing January 1998

ISBN 0-915099-98-5

The Health Answer Book: The Complete Guide to Symptoms, Causes, and Natural Cures for Hundreds of Health Problems

This book is for information only and is not intended to be a medical guide for self-diagnosis or self-treatment. It does not constitute medical advice and should not be construed as such or used in place of your doctor's medical advice. We recommend in all cases that you contact your personal doctor or health care provider before taking or discontinuing any medication, or before treating yourself in any way.

While every attempt has been made to assure that the information in this book is true and accurate, errors may occur; and it is not possible to cover every symptom, condition, and treatment. The publisher, editors, and technical advisor disclaim all liability in the connection with the use of the information in this book.

SPECIAL THANKS

The editors of FC&A thank Mark Anders, M.D. for his assistance with the completion of this project. We appreciate his concern for accuracy, attention to detail, and obvious dedication to providing quality health care.

"Consider it pure joy, my brothers, whenever you face trials of many kinds, because you know that the testing of your faith develops perseverance."

James 1:2-3

"I have told you these things, so that in me you may have peace. In this world you will have trouble. But take heart! I have overcome the world."

John 16:33

Contents

Alphabetical Listing of Conditions

Foreword

The Health Answer Book: The Complete Guide to Symptoms, Causes and Natural Cures for Hundreds of Health Problems is a new book by the fine editors at FC&A Publishing. They endeavor to provide sound, practical health information to adults of all ages. The writers have waded through an enormous number of peer-reviewed journals (research and reviews written by doctors for doctors), professional medical textbooks, pamphlets, and brochures to accomplish this goal.

The book's contribution to educating the lay person is commendable. Although it is designed as a quick reference book, you will benefit from reading the entire book, with its simple, yet captivating style.

Most of us simply endured mundane health courses before we graduated from high school. As we age, however, we have a fresh appetite for medical matters — and with good reason. Many of the illnesses and health problems that plague us can now be prevented. We also know that early treatment will frequently lead to a better outcome.

There is a great need to widely transmit general medical knowledge if we are to continue to enjoy the advances seen in health care during the past century. As we approach the end of the millennium, a well-informed public is essential to the effectiveness of our health-care system.

However, the body of knowledge in the medical world is complex and vast, and individuals have difficulty staying abreast. As you are reminded throughout the book, *The Health Answer Book* is not intended to replace your personal physician but to supplement your medical knowledge. Each chapter covers one prominent symptom. An attention-getting introduction is followed by a list of additional symptoms.

Guided through a range of diagnostic possibilities suggested by the particular group of symptoms, you are given explanations about what can be done immediately to correct the problem and what the long-range approach might be.

Perhaps for some time now you, or someone close to you, have been ignoring a certain nagging set of symptoms, or maybe you only recently developed a problem. Either way, this book arms you with information that can help.

Clearly, making the healthy choice to read the advice in this book should not only educate, but also translate into a higher quality and longer life.

Mark A. Anders, M.D.

How to use this book

Body language. It can tell other people what you are thinking or feeling just by a wink of your eye or a turn of your shoulder. But what if your body is talking to you — not to someone else? When you experience certain symptoms, such as a headache or dizziness, your body may be trying to tell you something is not quite right.

If you're like most people, you probably have a tough time understanding this type of body language. In that case, buying this book was a good decision. *The Health Answer Book* is full of information about symptoms, causes, and natural cures for hundreds of health problems — information that can help you figure out the messages your body is sending you.

For example, if you are having chest pain, does it mean you're suffering a heart attack or just an attack of heartburn? Do you need an ambulance or an antacid? With this book, you can set your mind at ease by simply turning to the appropriate section for the answer.

We've included many of the most common symptoms of health problems, arranged alphabetically so you can find them quickly and easily. Under each symptom, you'll find a list of conditions that could be causing your problem. Although we cannot diagnose your condition for you, we can give you a solid place to start looking for answers. And because we emphasize natural treatments, we also provide you with plenty of self-help tips.

Using the *It's time to see your doctor* section

This section helps you put the pieces of your health puzzle together. If you have a certain combination of symptoms, you should be able to narrow down your condition more easily. Under the *It's time to see your doctor* section, you'll find a list of possible conditions that could be causing those symptoms. These cover emergency and critical conditions, as well as others that may require a doctor's supervision. We listed these conditions for at least one of the following reasons:

❖ Not treating the condition could lead to something worse, possibly death.

❖ The condition could continue for a long time without improvement.

❖ A prescription medication may be necessary for treatment.

❖ Self-help measures alone might not provide a cure.

If you decide you need to see your doctor, based on the information you read in *The Health Answer Book*, you will be well-informed about your possible condition and better prepared to discuss it with your doctor.

Using the *Table of Contents* and *Alphabetical Listing of Conditions*

The *Table of Contents* tells you on which page you can find your symptom. For example, if your lower back hurts, or you're tired all the time, you would look up the headings "Back pain" or "Fatigue" in the *Table of Contents*. When you check those symptoms, you'll learn what conditions might be causing your problem.

If you want to know more about a particular condition, such as tendinitis or Alzheimer's disease, try the *Alphabetical Listing of Conditions* first. The darker numbers in this listing mark the pages where you will find additional information and self-help advice. For example, if you know you have carpal tunnel syndrome, look it up in the *Alphabetical Listing of Conditions*. You'll see a list of every page that carpal tunnel is mentioned. The darker page number will lead you to a more detailed explanation of this syndrome and ways to deal with or prevent it.

Using the *See also* references

Some conditions listed under the *It's time to see your doctor* sections are followed by *See also* _____. This also refers you to a section where that particular condition is covered in more depth.

The fact that you bought this book proves you are concerned about your health and want to make informed decisions about your health care. *The Health Answer Book* includes the most common health symptoms and conditions — the ones you deal with every day — and, in some cases, the ones most often overlooked by doctors.

We are confident T*he Health Answer Book* will provide you with a valuable resource for your most pressing health problems. We hope you'll use it often to help translate the signals your body sends you into a prescription for a happier, healthier life.

Abdominal pain, frequent

A cramping pain or spasm in the abdominal area

Everyone has abdominal discomfort now and then, but when those pains keep coming back, you need to find out what's wrong. You could be suffering from something as simple as gastritis, an inflammation of your stomach's lining, to something as serious as cancer of the stomach, liver, pancreas, or intestines.

 ### It's time to see your doctor if you have abdominal pain and:

- Nausea and vomiting
- Gas and bloating
- Jaundice (a yellow tint to your skin)
- Indigestion after eating fatty foods

If you have these symptoms, especially if your pain is located in your upper right abdomen or between your shoulder blades, you may have gallstones.

3

Gallstones are hard crystals, usually made up of cholesterol, that form in your gallbladder. (See also *Belching, bloating, and gas* chapter.)

- Intermittent diarrhea
- Unexplained weight loss
- Fever

If you have any of these symptoms, as well as spasms of pain in your abdomen, you may have Crohn's disease. The cause of this chronic disease is unknown, but the number of people who have it seems to be increasing.

- Rectal pain
- Blood or mucous discharge from rectum
- Abdominal cramping on your lower left side

These symptoms could mean you have proctitis, which is an inflammation of the rectum and the area around the anus.

- Loss of appetite (which may lead to weight loss)
- Cramping abdominal pain that is usually relieved by bowel movements
- Diarrhea alternating with constipation
- Nausea

These symptoms may mean you have irritable bowel syndrome (IBS). IBS is usually just an annoyance and does not cause any serious damage, but if it interferes with your lifestyle, discuss it with your doctor. (See also *Diarrhea* chapter.)

- Constipation
- Fever or nausea
- Tenderness in area over colon
- Blood in your stool

If you have any of these symptoms, you may have diverticulitis, an infection or inflammation of small pouches that can form in the walls of your intestine.

Protect your tummy from ulcers

Although stress and lifestyle can make ulcers worse, the main cause is a tiny, spiral-shaped bacteria called *Helicobacter pylori (H. pylori)*. These bacteria penetrate your stomach's protective lining, making it more susceptible to damage from digestive acids. They also cause your stomach to produce more acid, contributing even more to the development of a painful ulcer.

Your doctor can do a simple blood test to see if you are infected with *H. pylori*. If you are, he'll probably prescribe antibiotics to kill the bacteria, and he might recommend the following lifestyle changes.

❖ **Stop smoking.** Cigarette smoking increases your risk of developing an ulcer. It also makes existing ulcers heal more slowly and raises the chances that your ulcers will return after they've finally healed.

❖ **Can the coffee.** Many beverages and foods that contain caffeine, like coffee, tea, and colas, may cause your stomach to produce more acid than usual, making your ulcer pain worse.

❖ **Limit stress.** Although stress is no longer considered the major cause of ulcers, many people with ulcers say that emotional stress increases the pain. Physical stress, such as surgery or a serious injury, may trigger the formation of ulcers.

❖ **Don't overdo NSAIDs.** Nonsteroidal anti-inflammatory drugs (NSAIDs) can undermine your stomach's natural protection. Aspirin and ibuprofen are common NSAIDs taken for arthritis, headaches, or just minor aches and pains. If they are causing you stomach pain, ask your doctor about switching to another type of pain reliever.

Immediate help for diverticular disease

Diverticulosis is a condition in which pea-sized pouches form on the walls of your intestines. Although the small pouches, called diverticula, don't cause any symptoms themselves, they sometimes become infected and inflamed causing diverticulitis.

When a diverticulum becomes infected, bacteria can enter through tiny tears in your bowel, forming small abscesses. Sometimes these abscesses cause discomfort for a few days and then go away. In a few rare cases, the infection can break through the wall of the colon and spill out into your abdomen. This is a dangerous condition called peritonitis, which usually causes severe abdominal pain, fever, nausea, and vomiting. Peritonitis can lead to death if you don't get medical help quickly.

Although diverticulitis rarely becomes life-threatening, you should see your doctor. He will probably prescribe antibiotics to fight the infection. Bed rest and a clear liquid diet will help your tender bowels heal more quickly. You should also avoid eating small, hard foods like popcorn, nuts, and seeds because they can get stuck in an already inflamed pouch and irritate it even more. Surgery may be necessary to drain any abscesses that have formed.

The long-range plan for diverticular disease

If you're over 60, you have about a 50/50 chance of having diverticulosis. This common condition affects about half the people in the over 60 age group and about 10 percent of people over 40. Although the condition is common, complications from diverticulosis are rare. The best way to avoid complications is to avoid developing diverticulosis in the first place.

❖ **Fiber up**. A high-fiber diet can reduce your risk of developing those pesky pouches. Fresh fruits are especially important sources of fiber because they boost the growth of good microbes in your intestines. These tiny microbes help increase bowel movements and keep waste moving through your system rapidly, reducing your chances of developing diverticular disease. Many people who have diverticulitis find that their symptoms disappear within a couple of weeks if they simply add lots of fiber-rich foods to their diet. Some examples of good high-fiber fruits are blackberries, raspberries, blueberries, dates, and pears. Be sure you increase your intake of fiber a little at a time because a sudden increase may cause uncomfortable bloating and gas.

❖ **Wash it down with water.** When you're eating all those healthy fiber-rich foods, make sure you wash it down with a big glass of water. Water helps soften your stool so it passes through your intestines more easily. To help keep your digestive system running smoothly, drink at least eight glasses of water a day.

❖ **Trim the fat and red meat.** One scientific survey found that men who ate lots of fat and red meat were much more likely to have diverticular disease. Researchers think this may be because red meat causes intestinal bacteria to produce substances that weaken the colon, making it easier for diverticula to form. If you eat more chicken and fish and limit your fat, your intestines will appreciate it and so will your heart.

❖ **Schedule your bathroom breaks.** Constipation may make diverticular disease worse because waste sits in your intestines longer and builds up pressure that could weaken your colon walls. Schedule a regular time to go to the bathroom for a bowel movement. Don't strain when you go because that could also increase pressure on your colon.

Abdominal pain, sudden

A sudden cramping pain or spasm in the abdominal area

Abdominal pain can be caused by many things, from a mild case of food poisoning to life-threatening appendicitis. If your pain is severe and you have other symptoms, don't hesitate to get medical help.

☤ It's time to see the doctor when you have abdominal pain and:

- Nausea and vomiting
- Gas and bloating
- Jaundice (a yellow tint to the skin)
- Indigestion after eating fatty foods

If you have these symptoms, especially if your pain is located in your upper right abdomen or between your shoulder blades, you may have gallstones. Gallstones are hard crystals (usually made up of cholesterol) that form in your gallbladder. (See also *Belching, bloating, and gas* chapter.)

- Stomach pain, tenderness, or cramping, often worsened by eating
- Appetite loss
- Nausea, vomiting
- Gas, bloating

If you have these symptoms, you may have gastritis, an inflammation of the lining of your stomach. If symptoms are caused by a virus or a food you've eaten, they will normally disappear within two to three days. If they don't, see your doctor. (See also *Appetite loss* chapter.)

- Nausea and vomiting
- Flushed or pale skin
- Respiratory distress (coughing, wheezing, breathlessness)
- Itching
- Diarrhea

These symptoms may indicate that you have a food allergy. Keeping a food diary will help you identify potential culprits, and eliminating those foods may be the only treatment you need. If you are having breathing difficulty or if you pass out, you need medical help. A serious allergic reaction, known as anaphylaxis, can be fatal.

- Loss of appetite
- Nausea and vomiting
- Mild fever
- Severe constipation

If your abdominal pain is relieved by drawing your right thigh up while lying still, and you have the above symptoms, you may have appendicitis.

- Vaginal discharge
- Irregular bleeding
- Nausea and vomiting
- Fever

If you're a woman, the above symptoms may indicate that your abdominal pain is caused by pelvic inflammatory disease (PID).

- Vomiting
- Stomach pain
- Diarrhea (sometimes bloody)
- Other people who ate the same food as you also get sick

You may have food poisoning. Symptoms can begin as soon as one hour after eating contaminated food or as long as three to five days after eating the offending meal. Although most cases of food poisoning will run their course without serious complications, severe cases should be treated by a doctor.

Immediate help for food poisoning

Food poisoning affects about 7 million people in the United States each year. The symptoms include nausea, cramps, diarrhea, and in extreme cases, shock and collapse.

The most common cause of food poisoning is *Salmonella,* a type of bacteria found in farm animals, especially poultry.

Seafood can be particularly dangerous, especially if you eat it raw. Seafood that comes from warm waters may have bacteria called *Vibrio vulnificus*. People with liver disease, diabetes, AIDS, or cancer are more likely to get sick from this type of bacteria. For these people, eating raw shellfish can lead to death from blood poisoning. Heat destroys *Vibrio*, so avoid eating raw or undercooked seafood.

Most bacteria are destroyed by cooking, but some bacteria create toxins that can survive even high temperatures. The life-threatening botulism causes this rare type of food poisoning. Botulism is associated with home-canned foods that aren't processed properly. If you have difficulty speaking, visual disturbances, or muscle paralysis, in addition to vomiting, you may have botulism. See a doctor immediately.

Less severe cases of food poisoning can be treated at home, but if you have severe symptoms, see your doctor. Taking a sample of the suspected food with you might help your doctor identify the cause of your food poisoning and possibly prevent a widespread outbreak.

The long-range plan to prevent food poisoning

Follow this guide for safe food handling, from shopping to storing leftovers.

❖ **Shop smart.** When you are running errands, go grocery shopping last, and take your groceries straight home. Put them away immediately. Never leave food in a hot car. Check the expiration date on all food you buy. If you don't think you'll use it by the expiration date, don't buy it. Make sure the frozen foods you buy are frozen solid, and don't buy canned goods with dents, cracks, or bulging lids.

❖ **Store it safely.** An inexpensive thermometer could help protect you against food poisoning. Put one in your refrigerator and one in your freezer. The temperature of your refrigerator should not be above 40 degrees, and your freezer should remain at 0 degrees or less. Freeze fresh meat, poultry, or fish if you're not going to cook them within a few days. Thaw frozen foods in the refrigerator. Never thaw a package of meat at room temperature.

❖ **Keep it clean.** The bacteria that cause food poisoning hate a clean kitchen and clean hands. Wash your hands thoroughly with soap and warm water before you begin to prepare food. The juices from raw meat, fish, and poultry may contain bacteria, so keep them away from other foods. For example, if you chop up your chicken on a cutting board, be sure you wash the cutting board in hot soapy water before you chop your vegetables

Lactose intolerance

Millions of people are lactose intolerant. They are unable to digest lactose, a sugar found in milk. These people don't have enough of an enzyme called lactase, which breaks down lactose so it can be absorbed into the bloodstream. The most common symptoms of lactose intolerance are nausea, cramping, bloating, gas, and diarrhea.

Lactose intolerance is easy to treat — avoid foods that contain lactose. However, different people can tolerate different amounts of lactose, so you may not have to cut out dairy products altogether. Some people can tolerate aged cheeses and ice cream, but not other dairy products. You just have to experiment to see what your body can handle.

If you just love moo juice, try lactase enzymes. They're available without a prescription. One type is a liquid that you put in your milk container and wait 24 hours. This reduces the amount of lactose in your milk so you can digest it more easily. Another type is a chewable tablet that you take just before meals or snacks. You can also find many forms of lactose-reduced products in your supermarket.

When you limit your intake of dairy products, you need to be particularly careful that you get enough calcium. Green vegetables, like broccoli and collard greens, and fish, like sardines and salmon, are also good sources of calcium.

on it. It's also a good idea to rinse the cutting board in a mild bleach solution to thoroughly disinfect it. Remember that bacteria can live in the dishcloth or sponge you use to wash that cutting board. Be sure you wash your dishcloths and towels often and replace your sponges regularly.

❖ **Cook food thoroughly.** Eating your steaks and hamburgers rare increases your risk of food poisoning. For safety's sake, red meat should be cooked to 160 degrees and have no pink in the middle. Poultry should be cooked to 180 degrees, and the juices should run clear. *Salmonella* loves to lurk in eggs, so cook them until the yolk and the white are firm, not runny. Don't use recipes that call for uncooked eggs, and don't be tempted to sample that cookie dough or cake batter containing raw eggs. Wait until the goodies are baked to be safe.

❖ **Microwave magic.** Microwaves can make your life easier by cooking your food quickly and usually safely, but they sometimes leave cold spots in food that could harbor bacteria. To help eliminate these cold spots, cover your food with a lid or plastic wrap so the steam can help cook the food more evenly. Make sure your cover is vented, and don't let plastic wrap touch the surface of your food. If your microwave doesn't have a turntable, rotate your food once or twice during cooking. When a microwave recipe calls for standing time, make sure you let the food stand for the suggested length of time. Your food finishes cooking during this time.

❖ **Keep it cold.** Bacteria that cause food poisoning love warm temperatures. Don't leave leftovers out for more than two hours, and divide large amounts of food into several smaller containers so they will cool more quickly. If you're having a party that requires food be out for long periods of time, keep it on ice. Pack lunches in insulated carriers with a cold pack. Keep picnic food in an ice cooler, and try to keep your food out of the sun.

❖ **Lose those leftovers.** Leftovers may be thrifty, but they can also be dangerous. If you don't use food within a few days after you cook it, throw it out. Never taste food that looks or smells bad to see if it's still edible. It's not worth the risk. And while you can save some hard cheeses and salami that have mold on them by simply cutting off the moldy part, mold is usually an indication that the food is crawling with bacteria. Give it the old heave ho.

Ankle swelling

Puffiness around the ankle

"My feet are killing me!" Why does it seem that when our feet or ankles hurt, our entire day is ruined? In fact, foot and ankle problems profoundly affect our general health and sense of well-being. And because so much stress is placed on the tiny bones and network of muscles, tendons, and tissues in our ankles, injury is common.

Many times our ankles will swell for simple, easily explained reasons. If you have just ridden for several hours in the car or on an airplane, you may find your feet and ankles are swollen. In this case, there is no medical problem. Next time you travel, simply try to move about more frequently and elevate your legs if possible. The problem should not last for more than 48 hours. But sometimes, ankle swelling can mean something more serious.

⚕ It's time to see your doctor if you have ankle swelling and:

- Joint pain
- Redness and warmth in the joint

13

These could be the warning signs of arthritis, an inflammation of the cartilage and lining of the joints. Because the foot and ankle region has so many joints (33 to be exact), it is particularly vulnerable to arthritis. And remember, people over 50 are at higher risk. Don't put off seeing your doctor. Although arthritis cannot be cured, it can be treated; but if left unattended, the disease can become disabling. (See also *Joint pain* chapter.)

   Take a prescription or non-prescription drug
Consult a doctor on possible side effects or reactions to any drugs you are taking.

   A recent injury to your ankle
   Pain or tenderness
   Bleeding or bruising
   You can't put weight on your ankle
   Numbness, tingling or paralysis in your foot
   No pulse in your foot
It is possible you have fractured a bone in your ankle or upper foot. As you age, your bones become thinner and more brittle. Even a slight injury can break one of the small bones around the ankle joint. Don't delay seeing a doctor, especially if you are experiencing numbness, tingling or loss of pulse in your foot. If you break a bone, setting it becomes more difficult after several hours.

   Pain and a persistent itch in the affected area
   Distended veins in your ankles
You may not be experiencing an actual problem with your ankles, but rather a condition called varicose veins. This occurs when veins, usually in the legs, become swollen and twisted. They will appear larger and much bluer than normal. There are various causes of the condition, but few cures besides surgery. (See also *Leg pain* chapter.)

   Pain in the ankle, calf or thigh which does not go
      away with rest

14

- Tenderness and redness in the leg/foot area
- Pain when walking, raising your leg or flexing your foot
- Fever
- Rapid heartbeat

Sometimes after a long period of bed rest due to surgery or illness, blood pools in your veins, especially in the legs. If a clot forms within the veins of the lower legs and restricts blood flow, you may develop deep-vein thrombosis. Being overweight, smoking and taking estrogen increase the risk of this condition. You can help prevent it by giving up cigarettes, especially if you are taking estrogen; losing any extra pounds; and staying as active as possible even if confined to your bed.

- Shortness of breath or difficulty breathing, especially when lying down
- Fatigue or weakness
- A cough that is worse when you are lying down
- Wheezing
- Rapid or irregular heartbeat
- Low blood pressure
- Swollen neck veins
- Enlarged liver

These symptoms could mean you have developed a heart complication, called congestive heart failure, as a result of another disease or illness. High blood pressure, heart attacks, emphysema, or various infections can cause the heart to stop pumping as strongly as it should. Blood backs up into other organs, especially the lungs and liver, and these symptoms appear.

- Moderate to severe pain following an ankle injury
- Redness or bruising
- Difficulty moving ankle
- Difficulty putting weight on injured foot

You may have one of the most common injuries to the ankle: a simple sprain. This means you've stretched or torn your ligaments, the strong tissues attached to your bones. A sprain can happen any time the joint is stressed, usually if weight is placed on it at an awkward or unnatural angle. Sprains can range from mild to severe, and the pain can be slight to intense. If you find the discomfort is still quite strong, even after a couple of days, you should see a doctor or physical therapist.

Immediate help for a sprained ankle

If you are confident your injury is a sprained ankle, it is quite easy to care for it yourself. Here is a simple way to remember the four steps to follow when treating an ankle sprain: RICE:

❖ **Rest:** Walk as little as possible.

❖ **Ice:** Apply ice to your ankle for the first 24 hours after the injury. Place the ice in a plastic bag and wrap a thin towel around it. Hold the ice pack in place with an elastic bandage if you have one. If you can stand it, keep the ice on your ankle for 20 minutes, then off for 40 minutes. Repeat this throughout the day.

❖ **Compression:** Gently wrap your ankle with an elastic bandage in a figure-eight pattern. This means start the bandage on the ball of the foot, alternately wrap your ankle and your instep in a figure-eight, then continue wrapping a few inches up your leg. This will help keep the swelling down and support your ankle while it heals.

❖ **Elevation:** Keep your foot higher than your heart whenever possible. You should be resting anyway, so sit or lie down with your leg on several pillows. This keeps blood from pooling in the damaged tissues.

The long-range plan for a sprained ankle

A sprained ankle can take up to two weeks to heal, but that does not mean the joint will be as strong as it was before the injury. It's important that you give the tendons and tissues plenty of time to mend, strengthen the ankle with specific exercises, and take care not to reinjure it.

- ❖ **Don't rush the healing process.** Our bodies don't bounce back from an injury as quickly as they used to, so give your ankle lots of TLC. Stretch the muscles before you begin exercising them, rest, and wear sensible shoes.

- ❖ **Try an ankle workout.** It's important not only to regain strength and flexibility in your ankle, but to restore your balance and coordination as well. Even before you begin putting any weight on the ankle, massage the muscles and do a few ankle rotations. If you have access to the beach or a pool, take a walk through the water. This will help bring down the swelling and gently strengthen the muscles. Gradually work up to more strenuous exercises. Something like the toe-crunch is easy to do, even while sitting down, and it increases the strength in your foot and ankle. Lay a small towel on the floor, and place your foot on the short edge, with half your heel on the towel and half on the floor. Curl your toes so that the towel is bunched all the way to the arch of your foot. Start out doing this 10 times, gradually increasing the number until you need more of a challenge. Then place a soup or vegetable can on the end of the towel to add resistance.

- ❖ **Avoid reinjury.** Too often, people don't pay enough attention to an injury after the initial healing has taken place. You may think that everything is fine and return to life as normal. But if you've injured a joint that affects your movement you need to pay special attention to your home environment and daily routine. Check your house for areas where a weakened ankle could lead to trouble. Are rugs secured with some type of non-skid backing? Is there a hand grip for stepping in and out of the shower or tub? Do you have adequate lighting, both day and night, for trips up and down the stairs? If you end up on crutches due to an ankle sprain, this accident-proofing is even more important.

You or your doctor might feel you need physical therapy to complete your rehabilitation. Your therapist will work with you on specific exercises to increase movement in the foot; perhaps do a gait analysis, which studies the way you walk; and help you improve your general flexibility, balance, and coordination.

Anxiety

Feeling nervous, edgy, and worried

Feeling anxious about being anxious? Well, take comfort in the fact that you're not alone. More people in the U.S. suffer from anxiety than any other mental health problem.

However, this doesn't mean you should just resign yourself to always being anxious. Unchecked anxiety can take a serious toll on your health. According to Dr. Ichiro Kawachi, assistant professor at the Harvard School of Public Health, if you're prone to everyday anxiety, you may be as much as 4 1/2 times more likely to die of heart failure than people who aren't anxious.

Actually, anxiety is a natural healthy response that is part of your body's protective fight-or-flight response. Normal levels motivate you to do your best. However, if you're anxious all the time, you may have problems getting things done.

People with generalized or chronic anxiety typically feel constantly anxious for six months or more. Panic disorder is a type of spontaneous anxiety that can strike without warning and cause severe chest pain, difficulty breathing, and intense fear of dying or going crazy. Post-traumatic stress disorder is another type of anxiety triggered by a traumatic event that causes flashbacks or nightmares. Even phobias, intense fears of certain situations or things such as heights or spiders, are a type of anxiety.

Almost all types of anxiety are best relieved by addressing problems triggering the worry and fear. A reputable psychologist can help you understand and deal with underlying difficulties. To get the most help for your money, look for a counselor who uses behavior therapy and other methods to conquer your anxiety instead of just encouraging you to talk about it endlessly. Many excellent self-help books also are available.

 ## It's time to see your doctor if you have anxiety and:

- Sweating
- Clammy skin
- Chest pain, heaviness, or tightness
- Coughing, shortness of breath
- Nausea, vomiting
- Pain that radiates from the chest to arms, back, jaw, neck, or stomach

These symptoms suggest you may be having a heart attack. Call for help or go to an emergency room or hospital immediately.

- Redness, swelling, itching
- Wheezing or breathing difficulty
- Yellow skin or eyes
- Fever
- Joint pain

If you're currently taking prescription medicine or have recently received an injection, you may be having a reaction to the drug. Symptoms may occur within a few seconds or up to 30 minutes after taking the medicine. If you're having difficulty breathing, your reaction may become life-threatening, and you should seek emergency care immediately. For any other reaction, simply talk with your doctor as soon as possible. Although almost any drug can trigger a reaction, the following drugs top the list of troublemakers: penicillin and cephalosporin antibiotics, sulfa drugs, vaccines, allergy shots, and the iodine injections used for some x-rays.

- Unexplained weight loss
- Increased appetite
- Excessive thirst
- Frequent urination
- Fatigue
- Frequent infections

You may have diabetes. You will need insulin to control this disorder and should see your doctor immediately. If you delay, you could go into insulin shock, a medical emergency. (See also *Weight changes, unexplained* chapter.)

- Confusion
- Leg or muscle cramps
- Weakness
- Swelling

These symptoms suggest you may have too little or too much sodium in your blood. Since a sodium imbalance may signal an underlying disorder, see your doctor as soon as possible.

- Weakness and fatigue
- Unexplained weight loss
- Hyperactivity
- Rapid, irregular heartbeat
- Always feel warm or hot
- Bulging eyes

You may be suffering from hyperthyroidism, also called thyrotoxicosis, toxic goiter, or Graves' disease. This is a relatively common disorder caused by an overactive thyroid. It can usually be controlled by medication. (See also *Weight changes, unexplained* chapter.)

- Pale skin
- Weakness and fatigue

These symptoms could indicate you have some type of anemia, due to a lack of iron, folic acid, or vitamin B12 in your diet. (See the *Food, vitamin, and mineral chart* on page 351.)

- Erratic behavior
- Loss of appetite
- Extreme tiredness
- Have recently stopped using or cut back on tobacco, alcohol, or sleeping pills

Trying to give up tobacco, alcohol, sleeping pills, or other drugs commonly causes anxiety as well as a host of other unpleasant side effects. Because conquering any addiction is difficult, you'll most likely have the best success if you work with your doctor or a self-help organization.

- Breast pain
- Bloating
- Dizziness
- Irritability
- Swelling of hands, ankles, and face

These symptoms point to premenstrual syndrome (PMS) as the probable cause of your problems. Symptoms usually begin seven to 14 days before your menstrual period and will stop as soon as menstruation begins.

- Loss of appetite
- Poor sleep
- Stomach pain
- Symptoms occur mainly in one particular location — work, home, etc.
- Have recently undergone a major life upset or change, such as death in the family, job change, or new financial responsibility

These symptoms often signal stress, a common trigger of anxiety.

Immediate help for stress

Stress happens. And when it does it makes every single sad state known to man seem worse. A little stress may help you perform at your peak. More than that will

Obsessive compulsive disorder

Obsessive compulsive disorder (OCD) is another area where anxiety rears its worrisome head.

This type of anxiety centers around intrusive thoughts, such as needless counting or repeating, fear of germs, or fear of hurting someone. The obsessive thought often leads to compulsive behavior. For example, someone with a fear of germs may spend hours washing and rewashing his hands, neglecting his job and family in the process.

Even if you're prone to checking certain things (such as whether or not the oven is off) a couple of times a day, you're probably not obsessive compulsive. You should only seek help when the thoughts and compulsions become so insistent that they interfere with your normal life.

At least two different approaches can provide effective relief from obsessive compulsive disorder: antidepressants and behavior therapy. In fact, researchers from the University of California at Los Angeles report that behavior therapy can produce the same beneficial changes in the brains of OCD sufferers as drugs do.

At this time, however, most OCD experts feel that a combination of drugs and behavior therapy is the best approach for controlling OCD.

If you're concerned that obsessive thoughts or compulsive actions are interfering with your quality of life, consult a qualified therapist who has experience with OCD. Life truly can be wonderful and worry free.

just help you make a mess of everything. Here are some ways to relieve stress, at least temporarily.

❖ **Check for culprits in your medicine cabinet.** Prescription drugs such as asthma inhalers, or even over-the-counter drugs such as diet pills and decongestants, can cause anxiety-like symptoms and intensify stress.

❖ **Cut back on alcohol and sweets.** These items just make stress worse.

❖ **Consider caffeine carefully.** The role of caffeine in our diets is a controversial subject. Some people swear by it, and some shun it like the plague. Most people know that too much caffeine can make you jittery and irritable. But a new study shows that just a little caffeine may have the opposite effect. Researchers found that caffeine lowered tension while it increased feelings of happiness and calmness. When they tested participants on their ability to recall and process information and solve problems, they performed better with caffeine. So the next time you're feeling tense, sit back with a cup of coffee, or do like the British and relax with a nice, hot cup of tea.

❖ **Take time to walk and talk.** Physical exercise helps relieve tension, and talking with a trusted friend or family member is a time-tested way to work out problems. Doing both together just doubles the benefits.

❖ **Make the most of this moment.** Focus all your energy and attention on whatever you're doing or whomever you're with now. This technique helps replace worries with more pleasurable, productive feelings.

❖ **Breathe your stress away.** Focusing on some internal function, such as breathing, sends your body the message that you are safe and secure. This helps relax muscles, reduce blood pressure, and calm your nerves. Often, feeling stressed or anxious causes you to breathe shallowly from your chest, increasing fatigue and anxiety. To relieve stress, close your eyes and concentrate on slow, deep breathing that forces your stomach muscles in and out. Make yourself exhale completely before you take another breath.

❖ **Treat yourself to a mini mental vacation.** Close your eyes and transport yourself to a favorite place. Recreate all the sights, smells, sounds, and pleasurable sensations you associate with your favorite spot.

❖ **Wash your worries away.** Sit by a fountain or stream, take a swim, luxuriate in a warm bath or shower, or simply wash your hands and face. Water works wonders in relieving stress and worry.

The long-range plan for stress

Although stress is not normally considered life-threatening, it can be lethal. In fact, stress has been linked to a large number of different disorders, from depression to sudden death. Unchecked stress can even kill perfectly healthy brain cells.

The bottom line — if you want to live a long, healthy life, don't mess with stress. Get it under control as soon as possible. Here are some helpful tips.

❖ **Try to pinpoint the source of your stress.** If nothing comes quickly to mind, put your feelings on paper. This will often help you uncover any hidden conflicts that may be bothering you. Don't make yourself more anxious by worrying that someone may discover what you've written. Simply tear up and throw the paper away once you're finished.

❖ **Make it a habit to meditate, daily if possible.** To begin, simply focus your mind on one word, phrase, or sound that you repeat silently to yourself. Don't worry about completely shutting out all other thoughts. When stray thoughts wander through your mind, just don't focus on them enough to distract you from meditating. Start with a five-minute session and gradually work up to 20 minutes. Some people find it helpful to meditate twice a day. The purpose of this mental exercise is to give your mind a rest from anxiety-producing thoughts. Mental relaxation helps reduce stress.

❖ **Relax your body to relax your mind.** Alternately tensing and releasing all the muscles in your body, beginning with your face and working down to your feet, will relax both your body and mind. To begin, close your eyes and take several deep breaths. Now, beginning with the muscles of your face, focus on tensing and relaxing all the major muscles in your body. Practice this relaxation technique regularly. Once you become skilled at this technique, you can use it to produce almost instant relaxation in any situation.

❖ **Review the day for a refreshing night's sleep.** Unresolved problems do not make good bed partners. And everyone knows that a poor night's sleep can lead to even more stress. That's why it's important to take a few minutes before bed each night and replay the day's events in your mind. Let go of all the unpleasant things that happened during the day, resolving to handle things better next time. Savor the day's successes. Make decisions about unresolved problems. Write decisions down if you're concerned about forgetting. Take your body through the relaxation routine mentioned above. Now you're ready for a sound night of sleep.

❖ **Plan to make your dreams come true.** Knowing you are working toward things that matter most to you can minimize frustrations that build up when you feel trapped in a rut of daily routine. Here are two tips to turn your dreams into reality:

● Write down your important goals.
● Break big projects into a series of small steps you can work on every day. Want to change jobs? Make one phone call contact today. Want to travel around the world? Eat in instead of out, and put the money you save into your around-the-world account.

❖ **Laugh it off.** Laughing is probably nature's most perfect antidote for stress. Stress creates unhealthy changes in the body, such as reducing your immune system's effectiveness. Laughing counteracts those very changes. Having a sense of humor also gives you a sense of control over your situation, no matter how irritating or annoying it seems to be. To give yourself a laugh, look for the absurd in your situation. Take time to enjoy jokes, funny movies, and books. If something ridiculous happens to you, turn your experience into a funny story for friends to enjoy. As Bill Cosby quips, "If you can laugh at it, you can survive it."

❖ **Investigate your vitamins.** According to a new clinical study, being even slightly deficient in vitamin C and the B vitamins can make you nervous, irritable, and depressed. This test of more than one thousand people found that those who were generally healthy but were low in these vitamins also felt fearful, forgetful, and unable to concentrate. When these people took supplements of vitamins B and C, they began to feel better all over, with less nervousness and irritability, a happier mood, more self-confidence, and more inclination to be physically active. If you're feeling generally anxious and "under the weather," check your diet to see if you're getting enough of these vital nutrients in the foods you eat. If not, you might want to consider a supplement. (See the *Food, vitamin, and mineral chart* on page 351.)

❖ **Minimize stress with magnesium.** When stress goes up, your body's magnesium levels go down. Lower levels of magnesium often mean increased irritability. American College of Nutrition researchers recommend supplementing with magnesium when stress levels are high. (See the *Food, vitamin, and mineral chart* on page 351.)

Appetite loss

No desire to eat
Thought of food makes you nauseous

Almost anything can interfere with your appetite, from various ailments (especially viruses and infections) to gory monster movies. Drugs can do their dirty work on your stomach, too, even though they may be working wonders for other parts of your body.

The heart drug digitalis is one common offender. It slowly builds up to toxic levels and saps the appetite, leading to unexplained weight loss that many people have mistaken for cancer. Other medicines that can minimize your appetite include antibiotics, decongestants, and painkillers. A lack of important nutrients like vitamin B12 or zinc may have the same effect.

Anyone familiar with motion sickness knows it can make you think of food in less than friendly terms. Even emotional upset can wreak havoc on your stomach. Anxiety, boredom, depression, and tension are all great appetite suppressants.

 ## It's time to see your doctor if you have appetite loss and:

- Excessive thirst and urination
- Nausea, vomiting
- Low energy levels
- Constipation

Your symptoms may signal that you have too much calcium in your blood. This is an emergency. Get medical care immediately.

- Tiredness, weakness
- Yellow eyes and skin
- Nausea, diarrhea, vomiting
- Low-grade fever (less than 101° F)
- Pain or discomfort in upper abdomen

Liver problems are a likely source of your symptoms. You may have cirrhosis of the liver, viral hepatitis, or liver cancer. See your doctor immediately.

- Tiredness, weakness
- Darkening of skin, freckles, scars, and breast nipples
- Low blood pressure, causing dizziness or faintness when you stand up
- Vomiting, diarrhea

Your symptoms could add up to Addison's disease, a condition your doctor can control with hormone treatments. If you experience pains, feel faint, have low blood pressure, or a high or low temperature, get help immediately. You may be having an adrenal crisis, which can be fatal if not treated promptly.

- Are cold all the time
- Decreased sweating
- Chest pain
- Weight gain
- Sleepiness or trouble sleeping
- Depression or trouble remembering things

These symptoms might indicate hypothyroidism, or an underactive thyroid. Although hypothyroidism is generally easy to treat with thyroid replacement drugs, it can cause life-threatening complications in rare cases, so it is important to see your doctor. (See also *Weight changes, unexplained* chapter.)

- Weakness and fatigue
- Pale skin

These symptoms could indicate you have some type of anemia, due to a lack of iron, folic acid, or vitamin B-12 in your diet. (See the *Food, vitamin, and mineral chart* on page 351.)

- Stomach pain, tenderness or cramping, often worsened by eating
- Gas, bloating
- Nausea, vomiting

These symptoms suggest you may be suffering from gastritis, an inflammation of the stomach. If symptoms are caused by a virus or a food you've eaten, they will normally disappear within two to three days. If they don't, see your doctor.

Immediate help for gastritis

Even those people with the proverbial cast-iron stomach get gut-wrenching gastritis now and then. Whether it's mild or more severe, your stomach is quick to let you know something strange is going on down there.

Gastritis attacks can surprise you suddenly or they may develop as a chronic condition more slowly over time. Many different things can trigger gastritis, including a bacterial or viral infection, surgery, serious injuries, anxiety, overwork, spicy foods, alcohol, and even certain

Gastroenteritis: The bad bellyache

When your stomach sends signals that cause you to double over in pain or scurry for the bathroom, you've probably got gastroenteritis — commonly called stomach or intestinal flu. The bad news is this virus is easily passed from person to person without any direct contact. The good news is, it will be gone within 48 hours and sometimes only hangs around for 24. You can't do much but wait it out, but you can make yourself more comfortable in the meantime.

❖ **Rest, in bed if possible.**

❖ **Wash your hands frequently.** This will help you avoid spreading the disease. You'll be less likely to catch gastroenteritis in the future if you wash your hands after every bathroom visit.

❖ **Drink plenty of liquids.** Once you have stopped vomiting, take drinks like Gatorade to help restore your salt and sugar levels to normal. If you have diarrhea, drink clear liquids every half hour. Once it eases up, try beverages such as unsweetened fruit juices, weak tea, and clear broth.

❖ **Add solid foods to your diet.** After you've tolerated liquids for 12 hours, you can begin adding solids. Good choices include cooked cereal, rice, flavored gelatin, and other bland soft foods. You should be able to eat normally within two to three days. See your doctor if you do not improve within three days. If you had severe vomiting and diarrhea, or suffer from diabetes or kidney problems, you may need to be checked for dehydration.

drugs. The drugs most often responsible for a stomach upset by gastritis include aspirin, ibuprofen, and other non-steroidal anti-inflammatory drugs (NSAIDs), as well as anticancer drugs.

Sometimes, it's simply a matter of age. As you grow older, your stomach lining deteriorates, making you more susceptible to irritants or infections that leave your stomach swollen and upset.

Fortunately, there are a number of ways to control your gastritis.

❖ **Limit your food intake.** Restrict your diet to liquids the first day of the attack. Frequently drink small amounts of milk, water, or weak tea.

❖ **Relieve pain with acetaminophen instead of aspirin,** which will just worsen your stomach irritation. Sometimes, gastritis may even cause chest pain. To relieve your discomfort, drink 16 ounces of lukewarm water slowly and continuously. However, if your chest pain spreads to your shoulder, neck, or arms or you feel faint or short of breath, you may be having a heart attack and should get medical help immediately.

❖ **Begin eating after 24 hours.** Choose only foods you know you can tolerate. Avoid foods, especially spicy ones, that you know upset your stomach. If you can't really pinpoint which foods cause you problems, keep a food diary for several days to see if you notice any patterns.

❖ **Eat small meals on a regular schedule.** You're less likely to suffer a gastritis attack if you eat six small meals a day instead of three large meals.

❖ **Avoid alcohol, caffeine and smoking.** All of these habits will only worsen gastritis.

❖ **Discuss your medicines with your doctor.** If you are taking prescription NSAIDs, certain anticancer drugs, or other medicines you suspect may be contributing to your gastritis, ask your doctor about switching to a different drug. If that's not possible, ask if you could take your medicine with food, which may reduce its irritating effect on your stomach.

Generally, repeat attacks of gastritis are caused by smoking, overeating, or drinking too much. You should talk to your doctor if you are sure none of those habits are contributing to the problem, especially if you see no improvement after trying the above measures.

Arm, elbow, or shoulder pain

Dull ache anywhere along your arm
Sharp, shooting pain when you move your arm

Tennis players sometimes get tennis elbow. Swimmers get swimmer's shoulder. You may not be a professional sports figure, but you still can be plagued by the same type of arm, elbow, or shoulder pain. Often, your muscles or joints will ache because you've pushed them a little too far when exercising. You don't even have to be doing aerobics or pumping iron — a weekend gardening session can be just as stressful. If you fall, or overdo it with heavy objects, a strain or sprain can be the fruit of your labor. Although most aches and pains are minor problems that go away with rest, sometimes that little pain is warning you of a more serious problem.

 ### It's time to see your doctor if you have arm, elbow, or shoulder pain and:

- Chest pain
- Lightheadedness, fainting
- Sweating
- Nausea

31

Shortness of breath

These are the warning signals of a heart attack, but not every heart attack has all these symptoms. If you notice several of them, don't wait. Get help immediately.

You've injured it within the past 24 hours
The injured area is misshapen
You're unable to move it

It's possible you have a fracture, dislocation, or serious injury. Get medical treatment at once.

Wheezing
Chest pain
Unexplained weight loss
Weakness and fatigue
Persistent coughing

Together, these symptoms could indicate lung cancer.

Fever and chills

You may have an infection that needs immediate medical care. Lyme disease is one example of a bacterial infection that affects the joints.

Morning joint stiffness
Limited movement and dexterity

This could mean osteoarthritis, a condition where the cartilage in your joints gradually breaks down. Usually, you will feel an aching pain when you move or put weight on your joints. (See also *Knee pain* chapter.)

Tenderness and limited movement
Worse pain when joint is bent
Fever (sometimes)

Bursitis is an inflammation of the soft tissue around your joints. Rest, along with aspirin or aspirin substitute, should clear up the problem in a few weeks. But if the pain persists, see you doctor. (See also *Hip pain* chapter.)

- Swelling
- Warmth in affected area
- Muscle pain or tenderness that increases with motion

If you have these symptoms, you may have tendinitis, an inflammation of one of your tendons. It is often caused by an injury, or by repeating the same motion over and over.

Immediate help for tendinitis

You spent the day cleaning out your attic, and you're proud of what you've accomplished. The cobwebs are gone, the boxes are sorted and stacked, and you actually managed to throw some things away. Unfortunately, you also managed to set off a bout of tendinitis in your arms and shoulders.

Tendons are strong cords of fiber that connect your muscles to your bones or to other muscles. When the tendons become inflamed, you have tendinitis. Tendons are so strong that you may pull off a piece of bone rather than tear them when you get injured. However, they can be pushed too far, and the price you pay is pain.

❖ **Rest.** If you have tendinitis, you've probably already overdone it. Now you need to give those inflamed tendons time to heal. Don't make your problem worse by trying to keep working through your pain.

❖ **Put it on ice.** Ice may prevent swelling as well as deaden the nerves that help you feel pain. You can buy ice packs at the store, or you can make your own by filling a plastic bag with ice. Wrap a towel around your ice pack to protect your skin, and don't apply ice for more than 15 minutes at a time.

❖ **Heat it up.** If you already have swelling, heat may work better than ice. The warmth increases your blood flow which may speed healing. Heat also can be relaxing. You can use an electric heating pad, take a hot bath, or apply hot wet towels to the painful area.

❖ **Ease the pain.** Aspirin and ibuprofen can help reduce the pain and inflammation of tendinitis.

If you've tried the above recommendations and are still in pain, or if your pain is severe, your doctor may give you a steroid shot to help speed healing.

The long-range plan for tendinitis

You love to spend your weekends doing something physical. You work in the yard, play tennis, or spend hours swimming at the local pool. While this may be lots of fun, weekend-only activity can lead to repeated bouts of tendinitis. To keep pain from spoiling your weekend fun, practice a few simple rules of prevention.

❖ **Stretch it out.** Do some stretching exercises every day to keep your tendons strong and flexible. It is especially important to stretch before jumping into any type of strenuous exercise.

❖ **Take it easy.** Be careful when you exercise to keep from straining your tendons or muscles. Make sure you lift heavy objects properly. Even carrying a heavy shoulder bag, book bag, or briefcase can put a strain on your arm or shoulder.

❖ **Make it strong.** One of the best ways to prevent the pain of overexertion is to make sure you exercise regularly. If your arms and shoulders get plenty of use, sudden exertion is less likely to cause a problem. Make sure you are comfortable with the exercises, then gradually make them more difficult. If an exercise is causing you pain, ease up. Pain is a warning signal, and you should pay attention to it.

Don't let tendinitis or other arm pain put a crimp in your activities. A little extra care will ensure that you keep going strong all weekend and on into the week.

Back pain

A sudden sharp pain in your back
Low backache or stiffness

Back pain is one of the most common problems known to man, and it happens to almost everyone at one time or another. Whether you're helping your neighbor move that heavy table into his den, or finally hoisting those Christmas boxes into the attic, one wrong move can cause back pain to strike like lightning. Most of the time, it's just strained muscles or ligaments that will respond to a little tender loving care. But sometimes the pain can indicate a more serious problem that needs your doctor's attention.

It's time to see your doctor if you have back pain and:

Fever or painful urination

Having fever or painful urination with your back pain could mean you have a virus such as influenza, or a kidney infection.

Difficulty in moving your arm or leg
Loss of bladder or bowel control

You've recently had a fall or injury and can't move an arm or leg, or you suddenly have bladder or bowel problems. Don't move, and get someone to call your doctor. You may have a spinal cord injury.

A sudden sharp pain in one spot along your spine

If you are over 60, this could be caused by the bone deterioration of osteoporosis.

In women only
- Pain that worsens when you lift something
- Discomfort in your pelvis
- Pain with sexual intercourse

These symptoms could be due to uterine prolapse, a condition in which your uterus has dropped down into your vagina. (See also **Sexual pain** chapter.)

In men only
- Frequent, burning urination
- Problems in beginning the urine stream and emptying your bladder
- Fever and chills
- Achy muscles and joints
- Unusual discharge from your penis

These symptoms could point to an infection of your prostate gland, known as prostatitis; a sexually transmitted disease such as gonorrhea; or an infection of your urethra, the tube that carries urine from your bladder. (See also **Sexual pain** chapter.)

- Pain in the bones of your back
- Weight loss
- Weakness
- Fatigue

Together, these symptoms could possibly signal cancer.

- A sudden sharp pain down the back of your leg
- Numbness or tingling in an arm or leg

Pain, numbness, or tingling in an arm or leg, especially with back pain, may mean pressure or damage to your spine. This could signal a ruptured disk.

Immediate help for back pain

If you can rule out these serious problems, count yourself lucky — your back pain is probably a result of

Help for disk problems

If you've been diagnosed with a ruptured disk (also known as herniated, protruding, or slipped disk), don't panic. It doesn't mean your road to recovery will include a detour for surgery. Some people find relief without ever going near a hospital.

First of all, be sure you're drinking enough water. Water acts as a cushion for all the joints of your body, including the disks of your spine. If your back hurts, try this old-fashioned remedy first.

Exercise is another possible cure. When one of your disks is injured, it loses fluid. Exercise gets your blood pumping harder and actually pushes some needed fluid back into the disk. Rest a while when you need to, but then get moving again. Exercises to stretch and strengthen your back may help restore your disk and keep you out of the hospital for good.

Another option is chiropractic care. In two recent studies comparing different types of medical care for back pain, people were more satisfied with chiropractic than with other treatments.

If you do choose surgery, be sure to discuss your operation and recovery in detail with your doctor. New forms of micro-surgery can be done through a very small (one-inch) cut. A new study compared the recovery times of people who had this kind of back surgery. Those who went back to work after just a couple of days fared better and had fewer complications than those who rested for up to 12 weeks.

good, old-fashioned overdoing it. First of all, stop doing whatever caused the attack. Being tough won't win you any trophies, and you shouldn't try to work through the pain — your back needs a break. Here are some additional pain-relieving steps you can take right away.

❖ **Grab a pill and a pillow.** Taking aspirin or ibuprofen is a quick way to stop the pain. These over-the-counter painkillers not only attack the discomfort, but also have anti-inflammatory power to help shrink swollen, inflamed muscles. Relax by lying on your back with a pillow under your knees, or on your side with a pillow between your knees.

❖ **Cool it or warm it.** An ice pack and a gentle back massage may help cool your searing pain. Massage for seven to 10 minutes, repeating as often as once an hour. If heat soothes you better, treat your aching back to a warm heating pad. Just be sure to turn it off before you fall asleep.

❖ **Get some rest, and then get going.** A day of bed rest may be needed and deserved when your back is really hurting, but don't overstay your welcome. A recent study showed that back-pain sufferers who went about their daily activities got well faster than those who exercised or stayed in bed. Get up as soon as you feel like it, even for short periods, and resume your normal activities. But take things easy for a while. Save that tennis match for later when your body can bounce back as easily as the ball.

The long-range plan for back pain

Beware the "big three" culprits of back pain: lack of exercise, bad posture, and lifting and reaching incorrectly. One of these probably caused your injury. If you don't want back pain to become a constant companion, you need to work on these problems.

❖ **Fitness counts.** Overall fitness makes a big difference in the health of your back. Get out and pump up your heart by walking, biking, or swimming at least 30 minutes three or four times a week. Even a quick 10-minute walk is a good beginning. Before you know it, you'll be up to a half hour or more of healthy, back-strengthening aerobic exercise.

❖ **Lighten the load.** If you need to shed a few excess pounds, find a healthy eating plan and stick with it. That extra load around your middle puts a real strain on your back. Give it a break and lighten up.

❖ **Snuff it out.** You have tons of reasons to stop smoking, and now you can add your aching back to that list, too. North Carolina researchers found that smokers tend to suffer more low back pain from on-the-job injuries. Maybe it's the lack of oxygen to your back, or a nagging smoker's cough, but the puffing may contribute to your discomfort.

❖ **Straighten up.** Good posture not only makes you look younger and slimmer, it gives your organs a chance to work properly. It also strengthens your bones, muscles, and ligaments. It's like giving your back a helping hand.

It may surprise you to learn that the muscles in your abdomen provide some of the main support for your back. Keep them strong with this simple exercise: Pull your stomach muscles up and in, and stand up straight. Hold to a count of 10, then relax and repeat four or five times. Do this several times a day. It's amazing how effective this simple exercise can be. Before you know it, your stomach will be flatter, and your back will be stronger.

Practice good posture when you sit too. Slumping in a chair or on a sofa puts tremendous strain on your back. Try to sit comfortably straight. If your back begins to ache, relieve the pressure by putting one or both feet on a footstool or by getting up and moving around. A "lumbar pillow," available at medical supply stores, or any small, firm pillow can relieve pain by supporting your lower back.

❖ **Baby your back.** Whether you're digging in the garden or scrubbing your kitchen floor, be kind to your back. Don't bend and twist at the same time. Keep your back as straight as you can, and move your arms and legs smoothly. Use tools with long handles to avoid leaning over.

To reach something on a high shelf, put one foot in front of the other and push off from your back foot as you reach up. Don't stretch your

39

Exercises for strengthening your back

The best way to prevent back pain and injury is to strengthen the muscles that surround and support your spine. Here are some basic exercises to make you resistant to back pain. Do your back workout at least three days a week, beginning with two or three repetitions and working up to 10 for each exercise.

❖ Lie on the floor with your knees bent and your feet flat. Suck in your stomach muscles and lift your seat off the floor. Let your back relax down, starting at the shoulders, and flatten it against the floor. Hold your back flat against the floor for a count of five and then relax.

❖ Beginning in the same position, fold your arms across your chest. Lift your head and shoulders slowly off the floor to a 45-degree angle, trying to feel the pull in your stomach muscles, not your neck. Hold for a count of five, then relax.

❖ Lie flat on your back with both legs out straight. Grab one knee and pull it straight back toward your chest. Point your foot toward your head. Hold for a count of five, then repeat with the other leg.

❖ Lie flat on your back with both knees bent. Lift one leg toward the ceiling with your knee straight and your foot pointed toward your head. Stretch your leg as far as possible over your head, holding for a count of five. Relax, and repeat with the other leg.

back into an awkward position. If it's difficult to reach, use a sturdy step stool, or wait for a taller friend to get it. Don't try to lift heavy things above shoulder height.

❖ **Give yourself a little lift.** Don't bend over when lifting something from the ground, especially if it's heavy. Use your knees to squat down, then let your legs lift the burden instead of your back.

❖ **Brace yourself.** If you do a lot of heavy lifting at work or at home, think "weight lifter," and get yourself a back brace. This corset-like contraption supports your back the same way a wide leather belt supports real weight lifters. In a California study of workers at large warehouse-style stores, back braces reduced injuries by one third.

❖ **Consider the stress effect.** Believe it or not, your mind may be the real problem when it comes to back pain. Are you having a hard time remembering how or when you got hurt? Do you ache in different parts of your neck, shoulders, lower back, buttocks, arms, or legs? Does the pain change from day to day or even hour to hour? If so, you may be suffering from TMS, or tension myositis syndrome. In his book *Mind Over Back Pain*, Dr. John Sarno says this pain is caused by emotional stress, such as anger or anxiety. Deal with your stress, says Dr. Sarno, and you will relieve your pain.

Every bit of time and effort you invest in caring for your back will pay huge dividends in return. Exercise, good posture, and a little tender loving care will keep the "workhorse" of your body fit and pain free well into your golden years.

Belching, bloating, and gas

Expelling gas from your mouth (burping)
A feeling of being uncomfortably full (of air)
Having an excess of digestive fumes

Having gas means constantly saying "excuse me." While little boys may think the expulsion of gas from their bodies is a funny thing, most adults find it extremely embarrassing. Though belching, bloating, and gas are usually more of an inconvenience than a medical problem — a sign that you ate too much cabbage or too many pinto beans— they occasionally can signal a more serious disorder.

 It's time to see your doctor if you have gas symptoms and:

- A recurrent, burning-type pain in your upper abdomen lasting 30 minutes to three hours
- Unexplained change in appetite or weight
- Vomiting
- Blood in stool

If you have this combination of symptoms, you may have an ulcer. Ulcers are small sores in the lining of your stomach or intestines. (See also *Abdominal pain, frequent* chapter.)

- Difficulty swallowing
- Acid-tasting stomach contents sometimes rise into your mouth when belching
- Burning, heavy, uncomfortable feeling in your chest or upper stomach

If you have these symptoms, especially if they get worse at night, you may have gastroesophageal reflux disease (GERD). This is a condition in which stomach acids back up into your esophagus and irritate its lining, causing the uncomfortable burning sensation known as heartburn. If you suffer from GERD for a long period of time, your esophagus can suffer severe damage, and even increase your risk of cancer, so don't just ignore these symptoms. (See also *Heartburn* chapter.)

- Nausea
- Diarrhea
- Abdominal cramps

These symptoms may point directly to your diet. Many people who are lactose intolerant have these symptoms because they cannot digest dairy products properly. (See also *Abdominal pain, sudden* chapter.)

- Loss of appetite (which may lead to weight loss)
- Cramping abdominal pain that is usually relieved by bowel movements
- Diarrhea alternating with constipation
- Nausea

These symptoms may mean you have irritable bowel syndrome (IBS). IBS is usually just an annoyance and does not cause any serious damage. But if it interferes with your lifestyle by keeping you away from public functions, discuss it with your doctor. (See also *Diarrhea* chapter.)

- Nausea and vomiting
- Severe pain spasms in your upper right abdomen or between shoulder blades
- Jaundice (yellow tint to the skin)
- Indigestion after eating fatty foods

If you have these symptoms, you may have gallstones. Gallstones are hard crystals, usually made up of cholesterol, which form in your gallbladder.

Immediate help for gallstones

If you swallowed a golfball, you'd probably consider that a medical emergency. But did you know your gallbladder may hold gallstones as large as a golfball? While most gallstones are much smaller, as tiny as a grain of sand, even the small ones can sometimes cause excruciating pain in certain locations.

How do these mysterious stones grow in your body? Your gallbladder stores bile, a yellowish liquid that helps digest fat. It's made up of water, cholesterol, fats, bile salts, and bilirubin, which gives bile its color. Bile is made in the liver, then goes to the gallbladder, which releases it into the intestines to do its digestive duty. Most gallstones develop when your bile contains too much cholesterol. The cholesterol accumulates and crystallizes into gallstones.

Sometimes you can have "silent" gallstones which you don't feel or even know about. The ones you do feel can make you want to scream out in pain, and will probably send you to the nearest doctor or hospital.

Small gallstones sometimes lodge in one of the ducts that lead to or from the gallbladder. If one gets stuck in the cystic duct, which carries bile from the gallbladder to the small intestine, it can painfully inflame your gallbladder. These stones also can lodge in the duct between the liver and the gallbladder, causing a bile duct infection. Symptoms include jaundice (yellowish skin and eyes), pain in your upper right abdomen, high fever, chills, clay-colored stool, and dark urine. If you have these symptoms, you should see your doctor immediately.

If you have a serious gallstone problem, your doctor may remove your gallbladder. Because it is just a storage area for bile, it is not a necessary organ. Without it, bile simply flows straight from the liver to the small intestine. Removing the gallbladder is the most common treatment for gallstones, so it is a fairly routine operation. Most people return to their normal eating and bowel habits within a few days after surgery.

Nonsurgical treatments are available which dissolve gallstones, but they may take months or even years to work completely.

The long-range plan for gallstones

You may or may not enjoy listening to the Rolling Stones, but you definitely don't want stones rolling around in your body and blocking up your digestive system. Gallstones affect about 10 percent of the population, and certain people are more likely to get them, including:

❖ Women between the ages of 20 and 60. Women are twice as likely to get gallstones as men.

❖ Women who are pregnant or use birth control pills or estrogen replacement therapy

❖ People who are overweight or lose weight quickly.

❖ Certain ethnic groups, such as Native Americans and Mexican-Americans.

If you are at risk for developing gallstones, try some preventive measures to stop them before they start.

❖ **Bulk up with fiber.** Fiber makes food move through your digestive system more quickly. It also binds with cholesterol to help eliminate the fatty substance in your stool so it doesn't return to your liver. This lowers your cholesterol level, and since most gallstones are made from excess cholesterol, it lowers your risk of gallstones as well.

❖ **Team up with water.** Drinking six to eight cups per day does your body a world of good. When your bile has enough water, it can easily dissolve the cholesterol that forms gallstones.

❖ **High C may help.** Although the jury's still out on this one, evidence seems to say that a lack of vitamin C makes you more likely to get gallstones. If you eat plenty of "high-C" foods, like citrus fruits, you may protect yourself from those nasty gall-bladder attacks.

❖ **Eat low-fat.** A low-fat diet is often recommended to prevent gallstones from forming.

❖ **Watch your weight.** Overweight people are much more likely to get gallstones. On the other hand, when you are losing weight, your chances of getting a gallstone actually go up. Sound like a no-win situation? The obvious solution is to keep your weight at a reasonable level from the start. But if those excess pounds do sneak up on you, try to lose them slowly. People who go on low-calorie diets to lose weight rapidly are the most likely to get gallstones. Besides, the more slowly you lose weight, the more likely you are to keep it off. If you think you are at risk for gallstones or want to begin a strict weight-loss program, discuss it with your doctor. He may decide you would benefit from ursodiol, a medication that can help prevent gall-stones.

Breast pain

A dull ache or stabbing pain in your breast

If you are having pain in your breast, perhaps you just need a better-fitting bra. On the other hand, your breast pain may be a side effect of a medicine that you are taking, or an indication that you have one of the conditions below.

It's time to see your doctor when you have breast pain and:

- Depression
- Irritability
- Headaches
- Swelling

This combination of symptoms indicates you may have pre-menstrual syndrome.

- Sweating, hot flashes
- Vaginal dryness
- Irregular periods

46

Depression, insomnia, nervousness

If you're the right age, these symptoms could mean you are entering menopause. (See also *Menstrual changes* chapter.)

Lumps in your breast
Nipple discharge
Breast swelling

These are the most common symptoms of fibrocystic breast disease.

Immediate help for fibrocystic breast disease

A lumpy mattress may make it difficult for you to sleep. Lumpy breasts may do the same if you are experiencing pain from fibrocystic breast disease. Fibrocystic breast disease causes round lumps in your breast which move easily within your breast tissue. They are not cancerous but are usually tender to the touch. These cysts often fill with fluid and may be either soft or firm. Discomfort may increase just before your menstrual period, as cysts enlarge due to changes in your hormone levels. In fact, some women find their breasts swell up so much that they have to wear a different size bra. Fortunately, the pain and swelling usually lessen when menstruation begins.

You can usually tell the difference between a fibrocystic lump and one that is cancerous. While a cyst moves within your breast tissue and may cause tenderness, a cancerous tumor doesn't move easily and usually causes no pain. If you have a questionable lump, however, see a doctor immediately.

If the pain from your cysts is severe, your doctor may prescribe medicine. He also could perform a needle aspiration to draw fluid out of the cyst. This decreases pressure on the surrounding breast tissue, giving you enough relief to perhaps sleep at night. That is, if you could just get a new mattress.

The long-range plan for fibrocystic breast disease

You may have longed for larger breasts when you were younger, but the pain and swelling of fibrocystic breast disease wasn't quite what you had in mind. If you suffer from this distressing disorder, here are some tips to shrink those cysts and ease your pain.

❖ **Cut the caffeine.** Cutting down on your coffee, cola, tea, and chocolate consumption may cut down on the lumps in your breast. The caffeine in

---

Breast cancer

One out of every eight women will find that the lump in her breast isn't fibrocystic breast disease — it's cancer. Breast cancer is the second leading cause of cancer deaths in women. But you can fight back against this dreaded disease and keep it from adding you to the growing death statistics.

❖ **Practice self defense.** One of the best ways to keep breast cancer from ravaging your body is to examine your breasts monthly, especially if you have fibrocystic breast disease.

❖ **See your doctor regularly.** You should have a breast exam every three years between the ages of 20 and 40. After age 40, schedule an exam every year. The American Cancer Society also recommends you get your first mammogram between the ages of 35 and 39, then schedule one every year after age 40.

❖ **Move it.** You can lower your risk of breast cancer by 60 percent if you exercise regularly. An extra 20 pounds can increase your breast cancer risk by more than 50 percent.

❖ **Use olive oil.** Harvard researchers found that women who use olive oil more than once a day lower their breast cancer risk by one-fourth.

❖ **Take an aspirin.** Research finds that NSAIDs (non-steroidal anti-inflammatory drugs) can cut your risk of breast cancer. Women who took aspirin or ibuprofen at least three times a week for five years cut their risk of developing breast cancer by one-third.

---

these products can contribute to the development of fibrocystic breast disease.

❖ **Slash salt and saturated fat.** High intakes of salt and saturated fat have also been associated with a higher risk of breast cysts.

❖ **Add some A.** Vitamin A has been shown to reduce the size of breast cysts as well as the pain associated with them in women with fibrocystic breast disease. One study found that 80 percent of the women tested who took vitamin A had a significant reduction in pain, and 40 percent reduced the size of their cysts by at least half. If you eat lots of fruits and vegetables, you should be getting plenty of vitamin A.

❖ **Try some E as well.** Another vitamin that may be helpful in warding off fibrocystic breast disease is vitamin E. Vegetable oils like corn, safflower, and wheat germ oil are the richest sources of vitamin E.

❖ **Make sure your bra fits.** A well-fitting bra that supports your breasts will help keep the tenderness to a minimum.

Breath, bad

Unpleasant, foul, or stale-smelling breath

Almost everyone has a case of bad breath, or halitosis, from time to time, usually due to spicy foods that smell wonderful on the plate but not so good on you. Most people understand this and will just stand a little farther away from you when you speak. But if bad breath is a chronic problem, that's a different situation. Not only can it affect your business and social life, it may also be a sign of illness that you shouldn't ignore. Bad breath that stays with you may mean you need your doctor's help.

It's time to see your doctor if you have bad breath and:

- Diabetes
- General weakness
- Nausea and vomiting
- Stomach pain and tenderness
- Rapid heartbeat
- Loss of appetite

If you are diabetic and your breath smells fruity and a little like acetone, the main ingredient in most nail polish removers, it could indicate a serious problem. Fruity-smelling breath could mean you have diabetic ketoacidosis, a dangerous condition in which your glucose level is severely out of balance. This is a medical emergency, and you should get help immediately.

- Stomach pain
- Itchy skin
- Fatigue and paleness
- Tingling, numbness, and burning in your legs and feet
- Muscle cramps and pain

If your breath constantly smells fishy or like ammonia, and you have any of these symptoms, you might have chronic kidney failure.

- A history of hepatitis, liver damage, or alcohol consumption
- Mild jaundice
- Mental confusion
- Poor appetite and weight loss
- Fatigue and weakness
- Nausea or vomiting of blood
- Excess fluid in legs or abdomen

If your breath has a musty, rotten-egg odor and you have some of the symptoms above, you might have cirrhosis of the liver.

Chronic cough with or without sputum
Shortness of breath
Fever and chills
Weight loss

Bad breath along with these symptoms may indicate a lung condition or infection, such as a lung abscess, bronchitis, pneumonia, or emphysema. (See also *Breathing difficulty* chapter.)

Painful joints
Extreme dryness of your mouth, eyes, vagina, nose, throat, and sinuses

Bad breath caused by extreme dryness of your mouth and nasal passages can be an indication of Sjogren's syndrome, an autoimmune disease common in people over the age of 50. (See also *Mouth dryness* chapter.)

Sinus drainage
Headache
Pain around your eyes and cheeks
A general ill feeling

Along with these symptoms, constant bad breath may indicate a sinus infection.

Teeth and gums hurt when you eat food that is cold, hot, or sweet
Intense pain when chewing on one side of your mouth
An unpleasant taste in your mouth

These symptoms could point to periodontitis (gum disease) or a tooth abscess. See your dentist as soon as possible to avoid complications such as tooth loss or an infection in your bloodstream.

Immediate help for bad breath

People have known for ages that a spicy lunch such as garlic chicken, liver and onions, or a pastrami sandwich, can give you "death breath" by afternoon. Even Shakespeare in *A Midsummer Night's Dream* said, "Eat

Drugs that can affect your breath

Bad breath can be a side effect of several commonly used drugs. If you are taking one of these drugs, don't stop without your doctor's permission. But if the bad breath is really bothering you or your family, ask if there's an alternative. Here are some drugs to watch for:

❖ Antineoplastic drugs, used to fight cancer, may cause mouth ulcers, bleeding of your gums, or a fungus infection in your mouth. Bad breath can result.

❖ Dimethyl sulfoxide (DMSO), used to treat bladder problems and muscle pain, gives you garlic breath. Your body actually breaks down this drug into the chemical essence of garlic, then excretes it through your lungs and skin.

Any drug or medical treatment that dries out your mouth can cause bad breath. If you've recently started taking a new medicine and have noticed that your mouth is dry and your breath is bad, the drug might be the cause. Here are some drugs that cause dry mouth:

❖ Anticholinergic drugs or drugs with anticholinergic effects include antidepressants (for depression), antihistamines (for allergy), antipsychotics (for schizophrenia and other mental conditions), antiparkinsonians (for Parkinson's disease), and some drugs for intestinal problems such as diarrhea.

❖ Diuretics, which remove excess fluid from your body, are often prescribed for high blood pressure and congestive heart failure. They also remove fluid from your saliva.

❖ Antihypertensives, used to control high blood pressure, can give you dry mouth and bad breath.

no onions nor garlic, for we are to utter sweet breath." Once the chemical compounds in the food get into your bloodstream, your lungs will excrete the odor. Breath spray or mints don't have a chance of covering it up.

Alcohol, coffee, and tobacco (either smoked or chewed) are also culprits in causing bad breath. And eating meat makes your breath more pungent than eating fruits and vegetables.

If you have an important appointment or plan a special evening with a loved one, choose something mild for your meal and avoid the problem altogether. Or try one of the new "internal" breath fresheners and see if it works for you.

Food and drinks aren't the only reasons for breath problems. Dryness, bacteria buildup, mild illness, and dental problems can also contribute. But you have plenty of ways to fight back and keep your breath smelling like a rose.

❖ **Start fresh in the morning.** While you sleep, your mouth is either closed and quiet or open and snoring like a buzz saw. Either way, it's drying out. Saliva has a natural cleansing action on your mouth, so when your mouth is low on saliva, as it is when you sleep, bacteria can flourish. That's the reason it's so important to brush your teeth well at bedtime, and it's also the reason you get "morning breath." Usually a good brushing and rinsing of your teeth and tongue will take care of the odor-causing bacteria.

❖ **Be firm but gentle with your tongue.** Your tongue is a huge source of bacteria and odor, so you need to clean it too. If brushing your tongue is too uncomfortable, you can use a special tongue scraper or the side of a spoon to gently scrape that sticky, germy film off your tongue. Either way, be gentle.

❖ **Avoid mouthwash and breath sprays.** Antiseptic and deodorant mouthwashes and sprays only cover up breath odor temporarily. The alcohol they contain throws off your mouth's natural chemical balance and dries it out, so using a mouthwash regularly can actually make your breath worse. Use mouthwash only if your dentist recommends it.

❖ **Up your intake of water.** Drinking water frequently will wash away bacteria and bits of food, helping to keep your mouth clean and odor free.

❖ **Eat regularly.** You're more likely to have halitosis when you skip meals or diet. Chewing stimulates the flow and the cleansing action of saliva in your mouth.

❖ **Try a sweet treat.** When you need to cover bad breath quickly, try something sweet or starchy. A sugary mint or a cracker or chip will divert the bacteria that cause bad breath.

❖ **Say "yo" to yogurt.** Eating yogurt or drinking buttermilk that contains active cultures will douse bad breath. The active lactobacillus bacteria make it hard for other odor-causing bacteria to grow.

The long-range plan for bad breath

Doctors estimate that only 10 to 15 percent of bad breath comes from illnesses that affect your whole body. The rest occurs because conditions go wrong inside your mouth. Here are some steps you can take over time to improve your oral condition and protect yourself from halitosis:

❖ **Take care of your teeth.** At a minimum, brush twice a day and floss once to keep your teeth in tip-top shape. Using a soft toothbrush and fluoride toothpaste, brush well along the gumline and over all tooth surfaces. When you floss, curve around each tooth to cover the side surfaces.

❖ **Visit your dentist.** Twice-yearly checkups and cleanings will keep you on track for a healthy, sweet-smelling mouth. If you have tooth decay or gingivitis (gum disease), both causes of bad breath, your dentist can find and fix the problem.

❖ **Improve your diet.** It takes a healthy body to maintain strong, healthy teeth. Emphasize fresh fruits, vegetables, and whole grains in your diet, rather than meat, fat, and sugary foods. You also need calcium to maintain strong bones and teeth. Skim milk and other low-fat dairy products are good sources of calcium. So are broccoli, spinach, cabbage, cauliflower, beans, and nuts.

❖ **Check your vitamins and minerals.** Deficiencies of vitamin A, vitamin B12, iron, or zinc may dry your mouth and cause tiny cracks that hold bacteria and food particles. A lack of vitamin C-rich fruits and vegetables can cause gum disease. The result in all these cases is bad breath. Be sure you get enough of the vitamins and minerals you need in your diet. (See the *Food, vitamin, and mineral chart* on page 351.)

❖ **Get a good rinse.** Prescription mouthwashes containing chlorhexidine seem to be effective in preventing gingivitis, or gum disease. In studies, this germ-killing mouth rinse reduced some of the bacteria in people's mouths by 50 percent. If you aren't able to brush and floss properly because of a physical disability, this rinse may help you avoid dental problems. If you're worried about getting gingivitis, ask your dentist if you're a candidate for this product.

❖ **Bring in a substitute.** For a person with Sjogren's syndrome, the condition known as xerostomia, or dry mouth, is a constant problem. If you have Sjogren's, ask your doctor about a saliva substitute that you take before meals. Chewing gum or sucking on a mint will naturally stimulate the flow of saliva and give your mouth some relief.

❖ **Deal with your dentures.** Dentures are a common source of bacteria and bad breath. If you have removable dentures, braces, or plates, keep them squeaky clean. Remove and brush them each night, then soak them in a disinfectant solution. Your dentist can tell you the best kind to use.

❖ **Try a little peroxide.** Watered-down hydrogen peroxide has been used for years as an antibacterial mouth rinse. Now research shows that putting peroxide in toothpaste may be an effective way to fight bad breath. A recent small study found that Mentadent, a fluoride toothpaste containing peroxide, reduced levels of odor-causing compounds

46 percent more than a regular fluoride tooth-paste. However, some health professionals are concerned that peroxide produces harmful free radicals which may cause cell changes in your gums. It's best to check with your dentist before using such products for long periods of time.

The quality of breath changes throughout life. A baby's breath has a sweet, delightful scent. There's even a delicate flower named after it. But as you age, the air you breathe out loses its sweetness and becomes less enticing. Changes in your salivary glands make your mouth drier as you get older, so your breath becomes more intense and not as pleasant. But don't be discouraged — it's just more important to keep your mouth as clean as possible.

If bad breath persists, see your doctor to rule out illness as a cause. Then try the tips above to keep your breath as fresh as a spring breeze.

Breathing difficulty

Feeling as if you can't take enough air into your lungs
Rapid, shallow breathing
Gasping
Tightness in your chest

When you think of "a breath of fresh air," you probably think of a new idea, a new outlook, or a new perspective on the same old things. It's something we all need once in a while. But an actual deep breath of fresh air is something you need many times a day. When you can't take that deep breath, it's frightening. But there is good news. Although many things cause shortness of breath, most can be treated and cured.

☤ It's time to see your doctor if you have shortness of breath and:

- Chest pain
- Pain spreading to your shoulders, neck, or arms
- Lightheadedness, fainting
- Sweating
- Nausea

A sudden shortness of breath along with chest pain may indicate a heart condition, such as a heartbeat irregularity or angina pectoris. But you may be having a heart attack, especially if you have these additional symptoms, so don't take chances — get medical help immediately.

- Sudden swelling of your face, hands, mouth, or throat
- Itching all over
- Wheezing, coughing, or sneezing
- Faintness or weakness
- Pounding or rapid heartbeat
- Numbness or tingling around your mouth

These symptoms indicate anaphylaxis, a severe allergic reaction. They can occur within a few seconds to a few minutes of your exposure to a substance you're allergic to. This is a medical emergency; loss of consciousness may be the next symptom to occur. If you have these symptoms, get medical help immediately. (See also *Wheezing* chapter.)

- Chest pain
- Cough, with or without bloody sputum
- Fainting or feeling faint
- Rapid heartbeat
- Low-grade fever

These symptoms, together with sudden shortness of breath, could indicate you have a pulmonary embolism, which is a blood clot in one of the arteries carrying blood to your lungs.

- Sudden shortness of breath
- Dizziness
- Severe, sharp pain in your side
- Symptoms of shock (rapid heartbeat, pale skin, extreme weakness)
- Cough and fever

These are the signs of a collapsed lung, which can be caused by injury, infection, tumors, surgery, or inhaling a small object such as a peanut.

- Headache
- Dizziness
- Faintness
- Nausea and vomiting

Carbon monoxide poisoning is caused by overexposure to carbon dioxide, usually from some kind of heating system, engine, or industrial fumes. (See also *Headache* chapter.)

- Fatigue
- Fever
- Irregular heartbeat
- Chest pain

When these symptoms accompany shortness of breath, they point to myocarditis or pericarditis, an inflammation of your heart or tissues around your heart. This condition can result from illness, surgery, radiation therapy, or a bad reaction to a drug.

- Shortness of breath or difficulty breathing, especially when lying down
- Cough
- Irregular or rapid heartbeat
- Weakness, fatigue, or feeling faint
- Swollen stomach, legs, and ankles

Together, these symptoms may indicate congestive heart failure, which is usually a complication of other illnesses such as heart or lung disease.

- Pale skin
- Weakness and fatigue

These symptoms could indicate you have some type of anemia, due to a lack of iron, folic acid, or vitamin B12 in your diet. (See the *Food, vitamin, and mineral chart* on page 351.)

- Persistent cough
- Burning or pressure in your chest
- Thick sputum that is difficult to cough up

These symptoms, especially a persistent cough and difficult breathing, could mean an inflammation of your lungs or air passages. If you work in a dusty place, you might have a lung inflammation such as asbestosis, silicosis, or pneumoconiosis. If dusty conditions are not part of your environment, it could be bronchitis, bronchiectasis, or chronic obstructive pulmonary disease.

- Fever and chills
- Cough with or without sputum
- Chest pain
- Stomach pain

These are symptoms of pneumonia, an infection that causes inflammation of the lungs.

Immediate help for pneumonia

Bacteria and viruses are the most frequent causes of pneumonia. An infectious disease by itself, pneumonia is also an all-too-common complication of other serious illnesses. When your defenses are low, you have a harder time combatting pneumonia germs when they invade. In fact, they can strike just when you seem to be getting better, and the blow can be lethal. In the United States, pneumonia is the sixth leading cause of death.

Pneumonia is difficult to diagnose in some situations. If you are elderly, you may not have the fever, coughing, and shortness of breath that go along with pneumonia in younger people. Visiting a doctor who routinely cares for older patients should ensure that he'll look at all the possibilities and diagnose your illness correctly.

Although it may seem unlikely, an unusual form of pneumonia can be caused by accidentally inhaling oil.

One woman contracted this type of pneumonia from applying petroleum jelly to the inside of her nose for several years to combat dryness. Other people have gotten this type of pneumonia from excessive use of lip balm or hand lotion.

If your doctor diagnoses your illness as pneumonia, he will prescribe either an antibiotic or antiviral medication to fend off the infection. You need your doctor's care for this illness, even though he may treat you at home instead of the hospital. Take his advice seriously and follow his instructions. You should be up and feeling better within a few days to a few weeks.

Here are some things you can do at home to speed your road to recovery.

- ❖ **Stay in bed.** Don't get up and about until your fever is gone and you no longer feel short of breath.
- ❖ **Use heat to treat your chest pain.** You may feel better with a warm heating pad or a hot compress (a small towel dipped in hot water and wrung out) against your chest.
- ❖ **Let the fluids flow.** Aim for drinking a glass of water or other liquid every hour. This helps to thin out the secretions from your lungs so you can cough them up more easily. Fruit juice is a good choice to nourish your body and keep up your strength.
- ❖ **Cool it.** Use a cool-air humidifier in the room where you're resting. Make sure it's cleaned every day so airborne bacteria that collect in the humidifier won't reinfect you.
- ❖ **Toss your tissues.** Have plenty of disposable tissues on hand to catch your sneezes and coughs, and dispose of them carefully so you don't spread the infection to someone else.
- ❖ **Keep on coughing.** If you're coughing up sputum, don't take a cough suppressant. You're helping rid your lungs of harmful secretions. If you have a dry, painful, non-productive cough, ask your doctor about taking a cough suppressant.

❖ Get some relief. You may want to take something for your pain and fever, such as acetaminophen, or a decongestant for your head and chest.

The long-range plan for pneumonia

The incidence of pneumonia has increased in recent years, especially in hospitals and nursing homes. Those at greatest risk include the elderly, alcoholics, recent surgical patients, and people weakened by chronic illness such as asthma, heart disease, diabetes, cancer, or lung disease. If you fall into one of these categories, try to avoid places and situations that put you at higher risk of catching this disease. Here are some tips to help you avoid pneumonia:

❖ **Don't procrastinate; vaccinate.** Ask your doctor if you should get a vaccination against pneumonia. It's a good idea if you're over 65 or have lung or kidney problems, cancer, diabetes, heart disease, or cirrhosis. A shot to shield you from the most common strains of pneumonia should be available at your local health department for a modest fee. One shot is usually all you need for a lifetime of protection.

❖ **Get your flu shot.** Although flu vaccines are not 100 percent effective, they can protect you against some strains of influenza. Flu is often the first strike that puts you at risk of pneumonia. It's particularly important to protect yourself from flu if you have diabetes, a weak immune system, or heart, lung, or kidney problems. Ask your spouse and close family members to get flu shots too, so they won't bring the flu to you.

❖ **Keep your distance.** If a friend or family member has a bad cold or the flu, don't get near them. Any respiratory illness puts you at higher risk of pneumonia. You don't want to hurt your dear one's feelings, of course, but you don't want to risk your health either.

❖ **Stay out of crowds** as much as you can during the winter months, known as the "flu season." Being in a large group of people increases your risk of getting respiratory infections that can lead to pneumonia.

❖ **Keep your hands clean.** Wash your hands frequently, especially after you've been around sick people or out in public. Your hands are a prime

---

How can you tell if it's pneumonia?

Usually it isn't difficult for your doctor to diagnose your pneumonia. But figuring out whether a bacterium, virus, or something more exotic is the cause of your problem is another story. Here are some unusual signs your doctor may look for:

❖ A blue tint to your lips, nails, or skin may mean you have bacterial pneumonia.

❖ As you recover from a cold or flu, you may experience one big chill before pneumonia symptoms set in. This means you probably have a simple infection that your own immune system can help conquer. If you experience several chills, you may have a complicated infection that has spread to some other part of your body. These may be caused by a streptococcus bacterium, a cousin of the bug that causes strep throat.

❖ If your mouth is full of fever blisters in addition to your other symptoms, it could be another sign of pneumonia caused by strep bacteria.

❖ If you live or work around a lot of birds or if you have a pet bird, you may have psittacosis pneumonia, which you can catch from breathing the air around an infected bird.

❖ Another type of pneumonia can attack people with bad teeth and gums. It is frequently a complication of severe alcoholism.

❖ You could have Legionnaire's disease if you have recently traveled on a cruise ship with a spa or stayed in a hotel where you used the spa.

---

gathering place for germs because of all the things they touch, such as doors, doorknobs, railings, shopping carts, and cash. Other people, some of them with respiratory infections, have touched these things too. Protect yourself by washing your hands the minute you walk in your door.

❖ **Douse the fire.** You probably already know the other health reasons to stop smoking, but you may not know it increases your risk of pneumonia. If you want to protect yourself from pneumonia and a host of other health problems, embark on a program to quit smoking.

❖ **Come in out of the cold.** It's just an old wives' tale that you catch a cold by being out in cold weather. But if you are already in a weakened state, breathing in really cold air can further stress your lungs and bronchial tubes and make you more vulnerable to pneumonia.

❖ **Bring down your stress level.** Some stress will keep you on your toes; too much can make you sick. A high level of stress will suppress your immune system so it can't do its job of fighting off disease. Give yourself a break and get rid of those unimportant things in your life that only stress you out.

❖ **Avoid pox like the plague.** Although it may seem to be only a childhood disease, it isn't. If you never had chickenpox as a child, you could catch it as an adult. It's a much more serious disease in adults, and pneumonia is one of the possible complications. If your little neighbor has a case of chickenpox, stay away until he's well.

❖ **Treat it right.** The next time you get a cold or other respiratory infection, be sure you do all the right things to treat it, and see your doctor early. Don't let the illness get out of hand and turn into a case of pneumonia.

Pneumonia is a serious illness but one you can easily protect yourself against. Your best defense is to steer clear of the hazards of winter illness. Follow our tips and do all you can to keep yourself healthy. If you get pneumonia despite your best efforts, follow your doctor's orders and take good care of yourself, and you should recover quickly.

Bruising, unexplained

Discoloration caused by blood pooling in tissue beneath the skin
No known injury
No broken skin

Life is one long contest — your body versus the world. As an adult, you may think you have put scrapes and bumps behind you, but age can bring a loss of coordination, diminished eyesight, and slowed reflexes. The resulting bruises can be surprisingly painful and slow to heal. But you have little cause for alarm if your encounters with the world are less than peaceful. It's only when bruises appear without any apparent cause that your situation needs closer attention.

 ## It's time to see your doctor if you have unexplained bruising and:

- Little or no urine
- Loss of appetite, nausea, and vomiting
- Diarrhea or constipation
- Headache, convulsions
- Drowsiness, irritability, or confusion
- Dry, itchy, pale skin
- Weak, irregular pulse
- Swelling
- Spontaneous bleeding

Acute kidney failure means your kidneys have suddenly stopped functioning. It usually results from another condition or illness. This is a potential emergency, and you should see your doctor immediately. You are at especially high risk if you have only one kidney or have recently had surgery or a severe injury.

- Fever
- Bleeding from nose or gums
- Fatigue
- Bone tenderness
- Headache, stomach pain
- Enlarged lymph nodes and spleen
- Repeated infections in your chest, throat, skin, or mouth

Leukemia is a type of cancer that affects the production of white blood cells. Your doctor can study a sample of your bone marrow to determine if you have the disease. Acute leukemia comes about more suddenly than chronic leukemia but has a fairly high survival rate.

- Red or purple spots on the skin
- Nosebleeds
- Bleeding in the mouth
- Blood in the urine
- Heavy vaginal bleeding
- Headaches or dizziness (sometimes)

Thrombocytopenia is a long word that means you don't have enough platelets in your blood. Platelets are the tiny disks that join together to stop bleeding. If you don't have enough platelets, your blood is unable to clot, so you bleed more heavily and often. There are many possible causes and treatments of thrombocytopenia, and recovery is high. You need to see a doctor for an accurate diagnosis.

- Fever
- Headache
- Weakness

- Pain in the bruised area
- General feeling of sickness

You may be suffering from an infection caused by a bacterium, virus, or parasite, or showing the first signs of several contagious illnesses.

- Swollen, occasionally bleeding gums
- Nosebleeds
- Loss of teeth
- Rough skin
- Weakness
- Hallucinations or odd behavior
- General aches and pains

These symptoms say your body is low on vitamin C. Also known as ascorbic acid, vitamin C helps maintain healthy bones, teeth, gums, ligaments, and blood vessels; fights infections and heals wounds; and helps your blood absorb iron. (See the *Food, vitamin, and mineral chart* on page 351.) (See also *Gum bleeding* chapter.)

- Abdominal pain, diarrhea, vomiting
- Small, flat, purple bruises appearing in patterns
- Affected area itches, prickles, or tingles
- Swelling in your joints or other places

This condition is called allergic purpura, or allergic rash. It is most often caused by a bacterial infection, but can be a reaction to drugs or certain foods.

- Areas affected are your thighs, hands and forearms

When the tissues that support the blood vessels under the skin age and thin, the blood vessels burst very easily. This is called common purpura and is widely seen in elderly women.

- Fatigue
- Bleeding from the nose, gums, rectum, or other areas
- Sores in the mouth, on the tongue or rectum

With these symptoms, you could be suffering from aplastic anemia, a condition where your bone marrow

does not produce enough blood cells. This is usually treatable, so see your doctor immediately.

Take a prescription or non-prescription drug
Bruising or blood spots under the skin could be a
reaction or side effect of any number of drugs.
Check with your doctor.

Blood spots under the skin
Unexplained bleeding from your gums, nose,
**   intestinal or urinary tract**
Slow clotting
If you lack vitamin K, you may show signs of these
symptoms. Certain bacteria in your intestines
make this vitamin, which the liver uses to produce
blood-clotting substances. Without enough vitamin
K, you will bleed more than usual.

Immediate help for vitamin K deficiency

If you suffer from cystic fibrosis, ulcerative colitis, or
chronic liver disease, or have had bowel surgery, you
may have a vitamin K deficiency. Eating right or taking a
vitamin supplement should be all you need to correct the
unusual bleeding and bruising. In the meantime, you
can help your body recover more quickly by treating it
gently.

❖ **Prevent unexpected bleeding.** Be especially careful
during your daily activities to protect yourself
from bumps and scrapes. Until a long-term remedy for the vitamin K deficiency kicks in, your body
is still open to bruising and bleeding. You should
take extra care when brushing your teeth, as your
gums may be tender and easily irritated.

❖ **Review your medication.** If you are on medications
such as anticoagulants or antibiotics, you cannot
make enough vitamin K. Anticoagulants are drugs
that prevent or delay blood clotting. Common
examples are dicumarol, enoxaparin, heparin, and
warfarin. Make sure you take only the required
dose of any of these drugs. Notify your doctor
immediately if you have any unusual bleeding.

Antibiotics taken over a long period may destroy the good bacteria in your intestines. Discuss other possible treatments with your doctor.

The long-range plan for vitamin K deficiency

❖ **Eat green.** If you have been diagnosed with a vitamin K deficiency, you should make a special effort to eat more vitamin-rich foods. Your doctor or a nutritionist can work with you on setting up a diet plan. Foods especially high in vitamin K are green leafy vegetables, especially lettuce, spinach, kale, broccoli, turnip greens, and cabbage; cauliflower; tomatoes; egg yolks; liver; pork; cereal grain products; fruits; dairy products, especially cheese; and vegetable oils such as rapeseed and soybean. (See the *Food, vitamin, and mineral chart* on page 351.)

❖ **Supplement.** Although it is best to get your vitamins and minerals from the foods you eat, sometimes supplements are required — especially if you have a serious deficiency. But remember, vitamin K supplements should only be taken under a doctor's care. He may give you something by mouth or as an injection, depending on your condition. Just to be safe, remind your doctor of any other medications you are taking.

It can be frightening to experience sudden bleeding and bruising, especially when you can't figure out what's causing it. But with proper treatment, you have a good chance for recovery. Sometimes, as with vitamin K deficiency, relief may be as close as the nearest grocery store.

Chest pain

Dull or sharp pain in chest

Intense pain under breastbone, radiating out to jaw, neck, or arms

Pain that increases when you breathe in or swallow

Pain ricochets through your chest. You clutch at your pocket, gasping for air. "This is the big one, Erma," you shout. "Call the ambulance."

Only to realize minutes later that you've got nothing more than a serious case of heartburn.

Chest pain is one of the scariest symptoms you can have, because its consequences can be fatal. Ideally, you are educating yourself ahead of time so you'll know whether your chest pain means "dial 911" or "no more of Mom's chicken cacciatore."

Heartburn is a heavy, warm, burning feeling in the chest, and it can feel remarkably like a heart attack. Heartburn may be caused by indigestion or by a hiatal hernia, which means the opening in your diaphragm where your esophagus passes through is weak and stretched out. That allows stomach acid to slosh back into your esophagus. Part of your stomach may even poke up through the opening into your chest.

Even if you're prone to heartburn, however, never hesitate to call the emergency rescue service when your chest hurts for more than a few minutes. Heart disease is America's No. 1 killer, and delay can be deadly.

⚕ It's time to see your doctor if you have chest pain and:

- Pain spreading to your shoulders, neck, or arms
- Lightheadedness, fainting
- Sweating

- Nausea
- Shortness of breath

These are the warning signals of a heart attack, but not every heart attack has all these symptoms. If you notice several of them, don't wait. Get help immediately.

- Sudden shortness of breath
- Severe, sharp pain in the side
- Dizziness
- Symptoms of shock (rapid heartbeat, pale skin, extreme weakness)
- Cough and fever

These are the signs of a collapsed lung, which can be caused by injury, infection, tumors, surgery, or inhaling a small object such as a peanut.

- Sudden shortness of breath
- Cough, with or without bloody sputum
- Fainting or feeling faint
- Rapid heartbeat
- Low-grade fever
- Recent bed rest because of injury, illness, or surgery

These symptoms, together with chest pain, could mean you have a pulmonary embolism, which is a blood clot in one of the arteries carrying blood to your lungs.

- Fever and chills
- Cough, possibly with blood
- Shortness of breath, difficulty breathing, wheezing

These are the signs of lung infection and inflammation — pleurisy, pneumonia, bronchitis, or blastomycosis. Blastomycosis is a fungal infection that starts in the lungs. You can get it from wood or the soil, especially if you're a gardener or farmer, or through a bite from an infected dog. Pneumonia is more common, but it can kill you quickly if you don't get antibiotics and proper treatment. Pleurisy is inflammation of the linings of your lungs, and it sometimes accompanies another disease such as pneumonia or congestive heart failure. Bronchitis affects your air passages, and it's usually accompanied by a low fever and chest discomfort or pressure rather than pain. (See also *Breathing difficulty* chapter.)

- Fever and chills
- Dry cough
- Difficulty breathing
- Tenderness over the heart and chest
- Throbbing heartbeat, irregular pulse

With this combination of symptoms, you could have pericarditis, an inflammation of the membrane around your heart. Your chest pain may spread to your neck and shoulder and get worse when you move.

- Fever and chills
- Several days of skin sensitivity or tingling along one nerve path anywhere on the face or body
- Burning or shooting pain along the affected nerve

You probably have shingles if you have these symptoms. Not that long ago, shingles weren't considered a medical emergency, but now we know you need to see your doctor immediately. A case of shingles that isn't treated quickly can do permanent damage to your nerves. (See also *Face pain* chapter.)

- Chest sensitive to the touch

Sharp, tight chest pain that gets worse when you move may mean the cartilage between your ribs is inflamed. It's called Tietze's Syndrome, or costochondritis, and it can be caused by an upper respiratory infection or an unusual physical activity. With inflamed cartilage, you would probably feel a sharp pain when you cough or bend over. The pain may be in more than one place, and it may radiate into your arm, just like pain from a heart attack.

A severe cough or an injury to the chest

If your chest pain is on one side and you've had a hacking cough, a recent fall, or a car accident, you may have a pulled muscle or a broken rib.

- Rapid, pounding heartbeat
- Difficulty breathing, shortness of breath
- Sweaty or clammy skin
- Stomach pain or nausea
- Overwhelming fears, poor memory, and concentration
- Blurred vision or eyelid twitching
- Fidgeting or irritability

Any combination of these symptoms, and many more, may mean you are suffering from severe anxiety or panic disorder. Stress, guilt, alcohol, drugs, or working too hard can cause anxiety and lead to chest pain. (See also *Anxiety* chapter.)

- Fatigue
- Difficulty taking a deep breath
- Throbbing or fluttering heartbeat
- Lightheadedness or dizziness

Most people with mitral valve prolapse never know they have it unless their doctor hears a murmur through a stethoscope, but some people have the symptoms listed above. The valve between your heart's left atrium and left ventricle doesn't close properly, and that failure to shut sometimes allows blood to flow back into the left ventricle. People who have this backflow usually have symptoms.

- Heavy tightness, aching, burning, or squeezing in the chest or between shoulder blades
- Difficulty breathing, or choking feeling
- Pain may spread to jaw or teeth
- Left arm, hand, shoulder or elbow aches, tingles, or feels numb and heavy
- Pale face and sweaty brow

These are the signs of an angina attack, a serious heart condition. The pain may go away quickly or last longer than 15 minutes, and it's caused by a lack of proper blood flow to the heart.

Immediate help for angina

Chest pain sufferers see a whole new meaning in Hawthorne's *The Scarlet Letter*. For you, the red A that burns the breast stands for Angina.

Angina is the likely culprit behind your chest pain if it isn't a heart attack or heartburn. Coronary artery disease causes angina, and the pain is a sign that your heart isn't getting enough blood (and hence not enough oxygen).

You can have angina when you are resting, but too much stress, too much to eat, or too much exercise usually trigger an attack. Your heart should be able to handle the added demand, but it can't when the arteries that lead to your heart are clogged (atherosclerosis). The blood circulation to your heart is enough for normal needs, but not enough when the needs increase, such as when you are running after a grandchild.

Here's what to do right away to reduce the pain:

❖ **Nix pain with nitroglycerin.** Nitroglycerin expands your blood vessels and can ease pain within seconds. Make sure you always have the chest ointment or the under-the-tongue tablets with you. If you know an angina attack is on the way (like before sex), you may want to go ahead and take a tablet. Ask your doctor for details about how much to take and when.

❖ **If it hurts, don't do it.** An annoying old gag, but good advice. You know what triggers your pain. Don't sprint after the bus; wait for the next one. Don't stuff yourself at dinner; save the dessert for later. When a remark makes your blood boil, count to 10 and live above the fray.

❖ **Decline the second glass of wine.** Too much alcohol raises your heart rate. That can bring on an attack.

The long-range plan for angina

Angina can be painful, but it does have a positive side. Unlike a heart attack, it doesn't cause permanent damage to your heart. And because the pain serves as a warning, people with angina tend not to have heart attacks, even though their risk is high. They don't overdo it, like a person with no built-in warning system might.

But because angina is the result of clogged arteries, it is undoubtedly a signal of heart disease. An attack can cause irregular heartbeat, which is occasionally fatal. Here's what you need to do to permanently reduce your risk of angina:

- ❖ **Get out of your recliner — nothing's finer for angina.** Regular exercise will prevent angina attacks caused by overexertion. Your heart actually grows more blood vessels to provide more blood to your heart. Activity only triggers angina if it's more than your heart is used to handling. Warm up indoors by walking in place or doing calisthenics before exercising in cold weather.

- ❖ **Sign a pact to stop smoking.** Smoking brings on angina for numerous reasons: Nicotine raises your blood pressure. Carbon monoxide in your bloodstream reduces the amount of oxygen your blood can carry. Cigarette smoke makes your blood stickier and more likely to clot.

- ❖ **Strive for inner peace.** Stress can immediately trigger an angina attack and raise your risk of heart disease over the long term. We bring most of our everyday stress on ourselves. We choose how we react to bad traffic, a bad boss, and bad news. People with ill family members, difficult marriages, and high-pressure careers must learn stress management and get outside help when they need it. Prayer, short walks, listening to your favorite self-help guru, and relaxation tapes can all de-stress your life.

- ❖ **Lower high blood pressure.** The lower your blood pressure, the lighter your heart's workload, and the less oxygen it needs. Eat a low-fat, high-fiber, low-salt diet; take your prescription blood pressure medicine; and avoid over-the-counter drugs (like decongestants) that raise your heart rate and blood pressure.

❖ **Take the weight off.** Many overweight people find their angina disappears after shedding a few pounds.

When you first experience chest pain, you need to visit your doctor, if not immediately call for an emergency rescue service. After you've been diagnosed with angina, report back to your doctor when you experience:

❖ Unusual or severe pain.
❖ Pain that lasts longer than usual or is unrelieved by nitroglycerin.
❖ Pain at a lower level of exertion than usual. For instance, walking fast on level ground now brings on an attack, and previously it took climbing a steep hill to bring on pain.
❖ Pain that wakes you up at night.

These are all signs of unstable angina, which you should take seriously since it can lead to a heart attack.

If you can, see your pain as a plus. Your heart has cried out its warning, and now you can make the critical lifestyle choices — diet, exercise, smoking, and stress — that will give you cardiac health and a long, productive life.

Confusion

A feeling of bewilderment
Inability to distinguish between things
Being unaware of time, place, or self

Feeling confused is a constant state for some of us. It seems we always have new technology to learn, different highway directions to master, or difficult forms to figure out. Confusion is not necessarily a bad thing; sometimes it forces you to dig for information until you find a satisfactory answer. If, however, you find that you are suddenly and unexpectedly muddled over routine activities, it could mean something more serious.

It's time to see your doctor if you have confusion and:

- Headache
- Blurred or double vision
- Dizziness
- Vomiting
- Fever
- Inability to speak
- Inability to move one side of your body

You suffer brain damage when your blood and oxygen supply is reduced or cut off to a portion of your brain. This is a stroke — a medical emergency. You may have different symptoms depending on how bad the stroke is and which artery it affects. Get help immediately. (See also *Slurred speech* chapter.)

- Nausea or vomiting
- Dizziness
- Severe headache
- Weakness
- Memory loss
- Loss of vision or visual disturbances

These symptoms could mean you have a brain tumor. If you start having seizures, get medical care immediately.

- Headache
- Dizziness
- Blurred vision
- Vomiting

If you notice these symptoms and have recently lost consciousness following a head injury, you may have a concussion.

- Insomnia
- Chest pain
- Decreased tolerance for cold
- Decreased sweating and appetite
- Weight gain or extreme thinness
- Mental problems like depression or poor memory

These symptoms might indicate hypothyroidism, an underactive thyroid. Although hypothyroidism is generally easy to treat with thyroid replacement drugs, it can cause life-threatening complications in rare cases, so it is important to see your doctor. (See also *Weight changes, unexplained* chapter.)

- Unexplained bruising
- Swollen, occasionally bleeding gums
- Nosebleeds
- Loss of teeth
- Rough skin
- Weakness
- Hallucinations or odd behavior
- General aches and pains

These symptoms say your body is low on vitamin C. Also known as ascorbic acid, vitamin C helps maintain healthy bones, teeth, gums, ligaments, and blood vessels; fights infections and heal wounds; and helps your blood absorb iron. (See the *Foods, vitamins, and minerals chart* on page 351.) (See also *Gum Bleeding* chapter.)

- Anxiety or mood swings
- Loss of appetite
- Difficulty sleeping
- Thoughts of death or suicide
- Feelings of sadness or hopelessness
- Lack of enjoyment in activities or life in general

Depression is a common condition, especially as you age. Physical problems, such as an illness, medication, or hormonal changes, can bring it on. So can social or psychological factors. Don't feel you have to fight it alone. Get help as soon as possible. (See also *Depression* chapter.)

- Memory loss
- Disorientation
- Anxiety
- Insomnia
- Lack of concentration
- Difficulty communicating and completing tasks
- Gradual changes in personality and mental abilities

These are just a few symptoms of Alzheimer's disease, a condition where your brain function gradually breaks down. Many treatable diseases, including depression, have the same symptoms as Alzheimer's, so get a thorough medical exam if you suspect this problem. (See also *Forgetfulness* chapter.)

- Extreme hunger
- Weakness
- Sweating, nervousness
- Headache
- Dizziness
- Rapid heartbeat
- Drowsiness

These symptoms could be caused by hypoglycemia, or low blood sugar. This means your body doesn't have enough energy to keep up with all its activities. The condition may result from diabetes, an over-active pancreas, a reaction to certain drugs, or even another condition. See your doctor for an accurate diagnosis. (See also *Faintness and weakness* chapter.)

- Headache
- Weakness
- Paleness
- Shortness of breath
- Sore tongue
- Depression
- Numbness and tingling in the arms and legs

You could be suffering from a vitamin B12 deficiency, also called pernicious anemia. Your body can't absorb vitamin B12, so the problem cannot be fixed by simple changes in your diet. You need to discuss it with your doctor.

Use a prescription or non-prescription drug

If you feel confused while taking medication, see your doctor immediately. You could be having a reaction to that drug.

- **Shivering**
- **Weakness**
- **Slurred speech**
- **Drowsiness**
- **Slowed heart rate**
- **Slow and shallow breathing**
- **Stiff, numb muscles**
- **Prolonged exposure to cold air or water**

If you are suffering from these symptoms, and your body temperature has fallen below 95° F, you may be a victim of hypothermia.

Immediate help for hypothermia

Older adults are at especially high risk of hypothermia. Your metabolism has slowed down, so it is harder for you to keep your body temperature normal when the weather gets cold. Your body also has lost some of its sensitivity to changes in temperature, so you may not even feel your body chilling. Since you have less body fat as you age, you lose heat more quickly. Finally, you're more likely to have another illness or condition, such as hypothyroidism or arthritis, that keeps you from fighting off hypothermia.

Imagine being caught in a thunderstorm and struggling to walk home in the driving rain. You're cold, wet, and physically exhausted — three conditions that can easily cause hypothermia. But most people are surprised to learn you can develop it even if the temperature is above 50° F and you're indoors. That's what makes it especially dangerous.

You are at highest risk if you work outside; are malnourished, homeless or a victim of some kind of trauma;

Hyperparathyroidism

You have four small parathyroid glands in your neck. They make a hormone which controls your body's calcium levels. Sometimes, one or more of these glands gets bigger or develops a small, benign tumor. When this happens, the glands malfunction, setting off a complex reaction in your body. Your blood ends up keeping too much calcium, and your kidneys react by getting rid of large amounts of calcium in your urine. This causes painful kidney stones.

The symptoms of hyperparathyroidism can include:

❖ excessive urination

❖ lower back pain

❖ general achiness, especially in your joints

❖ abdominal pain

❖ nausea and loss of appetite

❖ depression

❖ overall weakness

❖ confusion

Since different disorders cause this disease, treatments range from surgery to vitamin or mineral therapy to diet modification.

have been drinking alcohol; suffer from some type of mental illness; or become immersed in cold water. However, older adults that live alone are also at great risk.

If you suspect that you or someone else is suffering from hypothermia, seek a doctor's care immediately. This is a potentially life-threatening condition. If you must delay emergency room treatment, here are some first-aid guidelines.

❖ **Get warm — but slowly.** If the victim is outside, get indoors if possible. Take off any wet clothing and wrap the person in blankets. If necessary, use your own body heat to help rewarm her. But do not put her into a hot bath. The sudden heat causes blood to rush to the skin, away from the heart and brain. For an older adult, this could be fatal.

❖ **Pick your brew.** It won't matter if it is coffee, tea, or cocoa — just make sure it is warm. Don't force anything into an unconscious hypothermia victim.

❖ **Ban the booze.** Despite what you see in the movies, a gulp of brandy or shot of whisky are the worst things you can take to warm up. Alcohol dilates your blood vessels, which may make you feel warm at first, but only allows more heat to escape through your skin.

The long-range plan for hypothermia

Prevention is the best treatment for hypothermia. By planning ahead, you are better prepared to fight it.

❖ **Food is fuel.** Your body is a complex machine that needs the right combination of nutrients to keep it strong. Eating hot, nutritious food all winter will keep the cold at bay.

❖ **Check your medications.** Many prescription and non-prescription drugs can impair judgment, making it difficult to realize just how cold you really are. Of particular concern are sedatives, hypnotics, tranquilizers, and antihistamines.

❖ **Sweet dreams.** If you are tired, your resistance to practically everything is lower, so get plenty of rest.

❖ **Don't smoke.** You may feel warmer when you smoke a cigarette, but as with alcohol, it's not real warmth. Smoking actually narrows your blood vessels so that less blood circulates through your body.

❖ **Dress for the weather.** It is just common sense to keep your feet and hands warm during the winter, but do you ever think about your head? You can lose about 20 percent of your body's heat through your head because of all the blood flowing through your neck and brain. So always wear a hat, scarf, or earmuffs to keep your head warm. Make sure they're made of wool, acrylic, or the new "outdoor" materials. And remember to layer your clothing, even when you're indoors.

❖ **No singin' in the rain.** A wet chill can be more dangerous than dry cold, so always have a water-proof jacket available if you're going to be outside. Take special care if you participate in outdoor winter activities around water.

❖ **Set the thermostat.** Winter is not the time to skimp on your heating. You should keep your house at a temperature of at least 65°.

❖ **Stay active.** Indoors or out, you should keep moving. Avoid sitting too long at that park bench, and break up TV time with a few light chores or an errand. In this way, you can generate your own source of heat.

Hypothermia comes, just like the fog, on little cat feet, and, more often than not, will leave you unaware that your physical and mental abilities are shutting down. Practice good preventive wintertime habits and you won't get caught in the cold.

Constipation

Having infrequent, hard bowel movements
Straining during bowel movements

Having a bowel movement should be a natural, simple process. However, sometimes it seems to become a big production, with you anxiously trotting to the bathroom and then sitting there straining in vain. Does this mean you are constipated? Although many people think they're constipated if they don't have a daily bowel movement, that's not exactly true. According to doctors, you can truthfully claim you are constipated only if you have fewer than three bowel movements a week.

It's time to see your doctor if you have constipation and:

- Blood in your stool
- Black, tarry-looking stool
- Cramping stomach pain
- Unexplained weight loss
- Pain in the rectum

Although hemorrhoids can cause blood in or on your stool, polyps and rectum cancer also can cause bleeding. If you have any type of bleeding from the rectum, or if your stool is black and tarry, see your doctor. (See also *Rectal problems* chapter.)

- Decreased sweating, appetite, and tolerance for cold
- Chest pain
- Weight gain or extreme thinness
- Sleepiness or insomnia
- Mental problems like depression or poor memory

These symptoms might indicate hypothyroidism, an underactive thyroid. Although hypothyroidism is generally easy to treat with thyroid replacement drugs, it can cause life-threatening complications in rare cases, so it is important to see your doctor. (See also *Weight changes, unexplained* chapter.)

- Rectal pain
- Blood or mucus discharge from rectum
- Abdominal cramping on your lower left side

These symptoms could mean you have proctitis, which is an inflammation of the rectum and the area around the anus.

- Cramping abdominal pain
- Fever or nausea
- Tenderness in area over colon
- Blood in your stool

Diverticulosis is a condition in which pea-sized pouches form on the walls of your intestines. Many

83

people have diverticulosis and don't even know it because it may cause no symptoms. However, if those pouches become infected and inflamed, causing diverticulitis, you will experience the symptoms listed above. (See also **Abdominal pain, frequent** chapter.)

- **Loss of appetite (which may lead to weight loss)**
- **Cramping abdominal pain that is usually relieved by bowel movements**
- **Diarrhea alternating with constipation**
- **Nausea, gas, and bloating**

These symptoms may mean you have irritable bowel syndrome (IBS). IBS is usually just an annoyance and does not cause any serious damage. But if it interferes with your lifestyle by keeping you away from public functions, discuss it with your doctor. (See also **Diarrhea** chapter.)

Immediate help for constipation

If it's been a while between bowel movements, you may be tempted to reach for an over-the-counter laxative. While this may be good for temporary occasional use, you must be careful not to overuse them. You can become dependent on laxatives, and eventually your intestines become insensitive and no longer work properly. If you do decide to take a laxative, here is a guide to some common types.

❖ **Bulk-forming laxatives:** This kind of laxative works by absorbing water in your intestine, making your stool softer. Bulk laxatives include psyllium (Metamucil), methylcellulose (Citrucel), calcium polycarbophil (Fibercon), and bran. These are the safest kinds of laxatives, but they may keep your body from absorbing certain medicines.

❖ **Stimulants:** This kind of laxative makes your intestine contract. They can lead to dependency and can damage your bowel if you use them too much. These include phenolphthalein (Correctol, Ex-lax), bisacodyl (Dulcolax), castor oil, and senna (Senekot, Fletcher's Castoria).

❖ **Stool softeners:** These make your stool moister and prevent dehydration. They are often recommended after childbirth or surgery. The most common ones contain docusate (Colase, Dialose, and Surfak)

❖ **Lubricants:** These grease the stool so it slips through your intestine more easily. Mineral oil is the most common type of lubricant.

❖ **Osmotics:** These cause water to remain in your intestine, allowing your stool to move through problem free. These include milk of magnesia, citrate of magnesia, lactulose, and Epsom salts.

The long-range plan for constipation

Don't let yourself get weighed down by this uncomfortable condition. While constipation is occasionally a symptom of a larger problem, most of the time it is simply a sign of not enough fiber or water in your diet. Before you reach for the laxatives, try some of the following suggestions for eliminating your constipation.

❖ **Fill up with fiber.** Do you need to get some speed out of your bowels? One of the best and safest ways to get your bowel movements out of first gear (or park) is to eat a high-fiber diet. Fiber is the indigestible parts of plants. Since you don't digest it, it moves through your system more quickly. Insoluble fiber, the kind that doesn't dissolve in water, helps constipation by holding water in your intestines, softening your stool.

It's easy to add fiber to your diet. Just make sure you add it gradually, because a sudden increase in fiber may cause gas, bloating, or increased constipation. Try adding about 10 grams of fiber at a time until you eat about 25 to 30 grams of fiber daily. Your breakfast cereal can provide a great way to start the day off with a healthy dose of fiber. Some, like General Mills Fiber One, offer up to 13 grams of fiber per serving. Other good sources of fiber include whole-wheat bread, vegetables, fruits, and beans.

❖ **Bottoms up!** The simple task of lifting a glass of water to your lips six to eight times a day can make your trips to the bathroom much easier and more productive. Water helps soften your stool and move it more easily through your intestines. If you are also adding fiber to your diet, it is especially important to drink lots of water.

❖ **Move your body to help move your bowels.** Regular exercise will help keep you "regular." Elderly people who are bedridden are much more likely to become constipated than those who are physically active. You don't have to be able to run a marathon to keep your digestive process working. Mild to moderate exercise, like a brisk walk every day, is enough to encourage your bowels to move along.

❖ **Make it routine.** Just like babies, your bowels work much better if they are on a regular schedule, so try to go to the bathroom at about the same time every day. Mornings after breakfast are best, so pencil that time in on your calendar for a daily trip to the bathroom. Don't despair if your appointment isn't always a fruitful one. Remember, daily bowel movements are not necessary for good health. You just want to provide yourself with ample opportunities.

❖ **Sweeten the pot.** Honey has been used as a treatment for various ailments, including constipation, for centuries. Recent studies confirm honey's reputation as a laxative. Honey contains more fructose than glucose. While these are both natural sugars, foods that have more fructose are harder for most people to absorb, so they move through your digestive system faster.

❖ **Pay attention!** Your body tells you when it's time to visit the bathroom. If you don't heed these warnings and go, eventually you will become constipated. Consider it your body's way of paying you back for ignoring it.

Constipation may not be a life-threatening condition, but it tends to be the only thing you think about when you're suffering from a constricted bowel. If you get plenty of fiber and water, you can forget about having (or not having) a bowel movement and concentrate on something much more pleasant. Your life.

Coughing

A sudden expulsion of air from the chest
Dry, hacking, or uncontrolled spasms

Coughing may not seem helpful, especially when you've been doing it for days or weeks. It's annoying, it's tiring, and it's an embarrassing interruption in a church service or business meeting. But coughing does serve a purpose. Your body may use it to expel a bite of steak lodged in your throat, or irritating phlegm from an illness or allergy.

The cause of your cough may be as simple as a common cold, an allergy to your friend's perfume, or a reaction to the smoke in a restaurant. But it also could be a sign that something more serious is going on.

 ## It's time to see your doctor if you have coughing and:

Blood or bloody sputum when you cough
This is a symptom that demands your serious attention, no matter what other symptoms accompany it. See your doctor immediately.

Sudden shortness of breath
Pain in your chest
Fainting or feeling faint
Rapid heartbeat
Low-grade fever
These symptoms, together with a cough and possibly bloody sputum, could signal a pulmonary

87

embolism, a blood clot in one of the arteries carrying blood to your lungs.

- Shortness of breath or difficulty breathing, especially when lying down
- Irregular or rapid heartbeat
- Weakness, fatigue, or faintness
- Swollen stomach, ankles, and feet

These symptoms may be a sign of congestive heart failure, a complication of some heart or lung diseases.

- Wheezing
- Fever
- Fatigue
- Chest pain
- Unexplained weight loss
- Heavy sweating during the night

If you have a cough with sputum that continues to get worse, you may have a lung abscess, inflammation, or infection such as tuberculosis or bronchiectasis. These symptoms might also mean lung cancer.

- Breathing difficulty
- Fever and chills
- Chest and stomach pain

These point to pneumonia, an infection that causes inflammation of the lungs. Less likely but still possible is a fungal infection such as histoplasmosis, which occurs mostly in farmers, gardeners, and people who suffer a dog bite. You may have blastomycosis, another fungal infection, if you've handled soil contaminated with bird or bat droppings. (See also *Breathing difficulty* chapter.)

- Choking spells
- Fever
- Vomiting
- Extended fits of uncontrolled coughing ending in a high-pitched sound

88

You may have pertussis, also known as whooping cough — a contagious bacterial infection. Most people think of it as a childhood disease, but it's on the rise in adults as well.

- **Shortness of breath**
- **Burning or pressure in your chest**
- **Thick sputum that is difficult to cough up**

These symptoms, especially a persistent cough and difficult breathing, could mean your lungs or bronchial tubes are inflamed. If you work in a dusty place, you might have asbestosis, silicosis, or pneumoconiosis. In a dust-free environment, it could be bronchiectasis or chronic bronchitis. Bronchitis can attack year after year or become a permanent health problem known as chronic obstructive pulmonary disease (COPD).

- **Low-grade fever**
- **Burning or pressure in your chest**
- **Wheezing or shortness of breath**

If you have a cough that won't let up, which starts out dry then includes gray or yellow sputum, you may have acute bronchitis, an inflammation of the air passages of the lungs.

Immediate help for acute bronchitis

Your doctor diagnoses your symptoms of fever, shortness of breath, fits of coughing, and burning in your chest as bronchitis. If these symptoms are new to you, you probably have acute bronchitis, a condition that's harsh but doesn't last too long. It can come on suddenly after a bad cold or after breathing irritating fumes. Acute bronchitis usually lasts only a miserable week or two, though your cough can last longer. Here are some steps you can take to fight it.

❖ **Snuff out the smokes.** The most common reasons for getting bronchitis are smoking and breathing secondhand smoke. Continuing to smoke irritates your lungs and bronchial tubes and will make your bout with bronchitis last longer.

- ❖ **Fight the fever.** To reduce your fever and relieve pain, take acetaminophen.
- ❖ **Breathe easier.** Take frequent hot showers or stay in a room with a warm vaporizer to give your throat and chest some needed relief. Clean the humidifier daily so that airborne germs collecting in the moist atmosphere won't reinfect you.
- ❖ **Rest and relax.** Stay in bed until your fever is gone, and get plenty of rest even if you don't think you need it. The more you rest, the more quickly you'll get well.
- ❖ **Wet your whistle.** Every day, drink eight to 10 glasses of water, fruit juice, or tea to make mucus thinner and easier to cough up.
- ❖ **Eat well.** Nutritious food will help your body fight the infection. Eating junk food may be comforting, but it won't help you get over bronchitis.
- ❖ **Quiet your cough.** It's okay to take an over-the-counter cough suppressant, but only if your cough is dry (not producing sputum). You don't want to stop a cough completely, since this could trap mucus and germs in your bronchial tubes and cause more illness.
- ❖ **Declare war on germs.** Use disposable tissues instead of cloth handkerchiefs, which provide long-term housing for germs. Dispose of the tissues carefully so you don't infect someone else or reinfect yourself. Wash your hands frequently with antibacterial soap for the same reason.

Your doctor may prescribe a cough suppressant or expectorant to treat your cough. She might also prescribe an inhaler to open up your bronchial tubes and an antibiotic to fight bacteria.

Antibiotics are useful if you have a bacterial infection as well as bronchitis, but they don't treat the bronchitis itself. Ask your doctor if antibiotics are really necessary before you take them. If your cough begins to produce greenish-yellow sputum, you probably have a bacterial infection.

The long-range plan for acute bronchitis

Here are some additional steps you can take to avoid acute bronchitis in the future:

- ❖ **Shy away from smoke.** The irritation to your bronchial tubes and lungs makes smoke and smokers bad company for you.
- ❖ **Protect yourself.** Fighting off an illness or taking medication will suppress your immune system and lower your resistance. That's the time to stay away from people with colds. A case of acute bronchitis often begins with a simple cold.
- ❖ **Avoid irritants.** Your risk of bronchitis is much higher if you breathe fumes from acid, ammonia, or other lung-irritating chemicals. Dust is another culprit that can cause bronchitis.
- ❖ **Beware the chill of winter.** If you don't want your cold to become bronchitis, you should stay out of frigid air, an irritant to bronchial tubes. If you must exercise in really cold air, wear a face mask to warm the air before you breathe. When it's cold outside, don't sleep with a window open.

Immediate help for chronic bronchitis

Your doctor tells you your lingering cough means bronchitis. If you've had the illness two years in a row for as long as three months at a time, it's classified as chronic bronchitis. If you have chronic bronchitis, chances are you're a smoker.

That morning smoker's cough with lots of mucus can progress to a wrenching cough that stays with you all day, every day. If you catch it early, you can avoid emphysema and chronic obstructive pulmonary (lung) disease, frequent results of chronic bronchitis. But if you let the condition go too long without treatment, it can become a permanent health problem. It's wise to do all you can to keep chronic bronchitis from getting worse.

Whether you've had chronic bronchitis for two years or 10, here are some suggestions to help you feel better and be healthier:

- ❖ **Lower the smoke screen.** If you smoke or live with a smoker, you have to make a choice. The smoke

91

will make you progressively worse — you can't breathe smoke and be healthy at the same time. Your best choice? Quit smoking as soon as you can. Many products and programs are available to help you, and you'll feel better almost immediately.

❖ **Eat like a champion.** Poor nutrition makes chronic bronchitis easier to get and harder to get rid of. Here are some suggestions for a healthy diet to combat bronchitis:

- Go for whole foods. Fresh, unprocessed food is healthier and more nutritious than processed food. Choose whole fruit instead of fruit juice, whole grains instead of refined flour, and fresh vegetables, raw or lightly cooked.

- Avoid foods high in calories but low in nutrition. Soft drinks, fried foods, candy, sugary desserts, and fatty snacks fall into this category.

- Catch fish. Research shows that eating two and one half servings of fish per week may help prevent chronic obstructive pulmonary disease. Fish is a source of high-quality protein in your diet, too.

- Turn up the heat. Eating hot, spicy foods such as chili peppers, mustard, horseradish, cayenne pepper, garlic, and onions helps you feel better by opening your air passages.

- Get your vitamins and minerals. Make sure you are getting at least the recommended dietary allowance, especially of vitamins A, C, and E. Vegetables such as carrots, celery, watercress, and spinach provide these vitamins. Fruits such as grapes, oranges, lemons, and black currants are also good choices.

❖ **Take a nice long drink.** Drinking eight to 10 glasses of water or other healthy liquids a day will help thin mucus and make it easier to cough up.

❖ **Avoid allergens.** Dust, pollen, and harsh chemical fumes will irritate your bronchial tubes and lungs. Add a good filter to your air conditioning system to catch some of the allergens. Air pollution is a serious threat, so stay out of polluted air as much as you can.

❖ **Stay out of bad weather.** Cold, damp weather and freezing temperatures will aggravate your bronchitis. So will sudden temperature changes, such as going from a warm house to a cold car. Try to avoid extremes.

❖ **Play it cool.** If you laugh or talk loudly, cry, or get upset, it can trigger a fit of coughing. Tone down your activity and emotions to control your bronchitis.

❖ **Don't take cough suppressants.** For chronic bronchitis, you need a productive cough to get out the mucus.

The long-range plan for chronic bronchitis

Try these additional measures to prevent flare-ups:

❖ **Avoid colds and flu like the plague.** Even a mild cold can cause your bronchitis to act up. Wash your hands frequently to get rid of germs, especially when you've been out in public. Get a flu vaccination every year to prevent influenza, and ask your doctor if you should get a pneumonia vaccine as well. If you do catch something, have your doctor treat you right away.

❖ **Exercise for better health.** Regular aerobic exercise will not only strengthen and tone your muscles but will help reduce your shortness of breath. If you are overweight, as many people with chronic bronchitis are, exercise will also help you regain a healthy weight. Walking, riding a stationary bike, and stair climbing are good exercise choices.

❖ **Consider a big change.** Although it may seem drastic, the ultimate treatment for your chronic bronchitis may be to change jobs or move. Working around lots of dust or other pollutants will worsen your health. So will living in a polluted area or a climate with cold, damp winters. It may take a new job or a new state to improve your bronchitis. Just be sure to look before you leap. Visit an area with a warmer, drier climate before you move there to see if it makes a difference in your bronchitis.

The wrenching cough of bronchitis can be exhausting and discouraging. But along with your doctor's care, you have many ways to help yourself feel better. Probably the most important is to say good-bye to smoke and smoking.

If your bronchitis is still in the acute stage, "nip it in the bud," as Barney Fife would say, so it doesn't become a chronic problem. If it's already a constant companion, do all you can to keep it under control so you can feel better and live a healthier life.

Depression

Lack of energy
Sleep problems
Loss of appetite, or overeating
Boredom, no interest in doing things you used to enjoy
Headaches or chest pain with no physical cause

Lots of things can bring you down, from an unexpected dip in your bank account to a miserable cold your body is fighting. However, some of life's little surprises hit harder than others. Death of a family member or friend, loss of a job, divorce, financial upheaval, or a chronic illness commonly send many people into the downward spiral of depression. In fact, one out of every 10 Americans suffers a major depression at some point in her life. Although depression affects both sexes, it is more common in women.

Certain transition times, such as adolescence and middle age, are problems for many people. And for women, both postpartum depression and premenstrual syndrome (PMS) can send them plummeting into the depths of depression.

Drugs, especially tranquilizers or sedatives, can bring your mood down. Older people, who are more susceptible to drug side effects, may find that antihistamines, muscle relaxants, and antinausea medicines also trigger depressed feelings.

If, at any point, your depression interferes with your work or personal relationships, it's wise to talk to your doctor. It's possible your depression may signal some other disorder.

It's time to see your doctor if you have depression and:

- Unusually rapid, unexplained weight loss
- Pain in the back or upper abdomen
- Yellowing of the eyes or skin
- Nausea, vomiting

You may have cancer of the pancreas. See your doctor immediately.

- Chronic low back pain
- Upper abdominal pain
- Appetite loss
- Personality changes

You may be suffering from hyperparathyroidism, an overactive parathyroid, which causes a calcium buildup in your blood. See your doctor as soon as possible. (See also *Confusion* chapter.)

- Constipation
- Chest pain
- Weight gain or loss
- Sleepiness or insomnia
- Confusion, poor memory
- Decreased sweating, appetite, and tolerance for cold

These symptoms might indicate hypothyroidism, or an underactive thyroid. Although hypothyroidism is generally easy to treat with thyroid replacement drugs, it can cause life-threatening complications in rare cases, so it is important to see your doctor. (See also *Weight changes, unexplained* chapter.)

- Unexplained weight loss
- Increased appetite
- Excessive thirst
- Frequent urination
- Fatigue
- Frequent infections

You may have diabetes. Since you will need insulin to control this disorder, you should schedule an appointment with your doctor as soon as possible. (See also *Weight changes, unexplained* chapter.)

- Impotence
- Fatigue
- Irritability

If you are a man, you may be suffering from hypogonadism, sometimes called male menopause, caused by a lack of testosterone. This disorder may be triggered by stress, obesity, alcoholism, surgery, or certain drugs. See your doctor. If a blood test shows you do have a deficiency, testosterone replacement therapy will soon have you feeling like your old self again.

- Tiredness
- General muscle weakness and pain
- Low-grade fever
- Sore throat
- Forgetfulness, problems concentrating

Your symptoms could mean you have chronic fatigue syndrome. This disorder leaves you feeling extremely tired, although no one knows what causes it. See your doctor for treatment. (See also *Fatigue* chapter.)

- Weakness and fatigue
- Pale skin

These symptoms could indicate you have some type of anemia, due to a lack of iron, folic acid, or vitamin B-12 in your diet. (See the *Food, vitamin, and mineral chart* on page 351.)

Immediate help for depression

Everybody has ups and downs, but if you have more downs than ups, you may be depressed. Here are some quick tips that may pull you out of a slump.

- ❖ **Get plenty of sleep.** Even a slight sleep shortage can cause depression in some people.
- ❖ **Avoid alcohol.** Drinking alcohol regularly can slowly pull your body and mind into a state of depression. This effect may persist even on the days you don't drink at all. If you cut out alcohol, your depression will probably disappear in a few days. If you have trouble giving up alcohol, see your doctor. You may have an addiction that needs professional care.
- ❖ **Control your stress.** You can't always control the events in your life, but you can control your reaction. A calm, organized, logical approach to problems is better than flying off the handle or letting yourself fall apart.
- ❖ **Talk it out.** Just talking about your troubles with a counselor or trusted friend can make you feel better and give you a more balanced perspective on how to handle the problems in your life.
- ❖ **Relax.** Take some time for yourself each day, even if it is only for a few minutes, to physically relax your body and mind. Get involved in any activity that diverts your mind from everyday stresses and strains.
- ❖ **Sniff your blues away.** According to Dr. Susan Schiffman, professor of medical psychology at Duke University Medical Center, sniffing a pleasant scent will give your spirits a major lift. The reason? The area of your brain that registers smells also controls emotions. Sniff perfume, fresh flowers, or even an aromatic herbal tea for a quick mood lift. If you like flowers, try the fragrance of osmanthus or tuberose — a

study found they offered the best relief from depression. Hyacinth, Douglas fir, and muguet scents also work well.

❖ **Improve your mood with caffeine.** A 10-year study of 86,626 registered nurses showed that those who drank two to three cups of coffee a day were less likely to commit suicide than those who didn't. More studies are needed to see if caffeine actually prevents depression. Just keep in mind that, for some people, caffeine has a nasty letdown effect that is almost worse than a bad mood.

❖ **Laugh a lot.** On average, a six-year-old laughs 300 times a day, an adult only 15 to 100 times a day. Studies show that the more humor and laughter you have in your life, the less likely you are to feel depressed. So, go ahead, do whatever it takes to lift your mood — whether it's a slapstick movie, cartoons, books, or a night out with goofy friends.

The long-range plan for depression

Typically, depression occurs when a person has more frustration and anger than she can handle. Although these levels differ for everyone, unchecked frustration and anger can lower the number of chemical messengers in your brain — the neurotransmitters — and eventually lead to depression. Here are some tips to help you handle a long-term battle with the blues.

❖ **You are what you think.** You may remember that old cliché more along the lines of "you are what you eat." However, when it comes to controlling depression, what you think may be more important than what you eat. A recent study of 60 people showed that adding a positive twist to a negative thought improved self-esteem and relieved depression. For example, if you think of yourself as a chronic complainer, add the thought, "but I am working every day to have a more positive attitude." Repeat it to yourself several times a day. And try not to be so critical. Studies show that people who often criticize themselves usually feel

Hello St. John's wort, good-bye depression

For years, folk medicine has relied on St. John's wort to relieve depression. Recently, the scientific community took note, and studies have shown it provides effective relief for mild to moderate depression. It also seems to have fewer short-term side effects than other antidepressants.

One side effect appears to be increased sensitivity to the sun, so if you plan to be outdoors, make sure you bring along your sunscreen and sunglasses. Also, beware of mixing St. John's wort with other antidepressant or diet drugs, such as Redux or the diet combo commonly called "fen-phen." You may have a reaction.

The German Commission E suggests using no more than two to four grams of the herb each day. When buying it in capsule form, look for a standardized product. This means the manufacturer has measured the active ingredients. Herbs that are not standardized may not contain enough of the active ingredient to be effective.

If you take the herb as a tea, pour one cup of boiling water over one to two heaping tablespoons of St. John's wort. Steep for 10 minutes. The herb seems to be most effective when you take it every day for four to six weeks.

more depressed and get less enjoyment from life than those who aren't as self-critical.

❖ **Eat well to feel well.** Strive for a balanced low-fat diet. Keep a journal for several days to get a clear view of your eating patterns. You may find some of your food fancies contribute to your depression, such as eating lots of sugar or skipping meals. Try to eat small frequent meals that contain a balance of proteins and carbohydrates.

❖ **Keep a journal.** You may not even know why you feel bad. Writing can help bring your unconscious into contact with your conscious mind and resolve conflicts that are bubbling just below the surface. Even if you know why you feel down, writing about it can help ease your mind and may even reveal solutions you hadn't thought of before.

❖ **Get involved and stay involved.** Although this may seem like the last thing you want to do, diving into a hobby, sport, or vacation may be just what you need to relieve your depression. If you've been over scheduling yourself, try to cut back. Spending time with others can also help pull you out of a slump. Finally, follow your regular routine. This may relieve stress and help improve your mood.

❖ **Lift the weight.** When you're depressed, it often seems as if the weight of the world is on your shoulders. According to Dr. Maria Fiatarone, you can lift that load right off your shoulders — with weights. Her study of a group of older depressed adults revealed that 10 weeks of weight lifting led to a two- to three-fold drop in depression levels.

❖ **Work it out.** Regular aerobic exercise, like walking or running, also is great for preventing depression. People who exercise regularly are less likely to feel depressed than people who are inactive. So lace up your walking shoes and beat the blues as you pound the pavement.

❖ **Boost your B's.** B vitamins that is. Even a small deficiency of the B vitamins, such as niacin, folic acid, thiamine, vitamin B2, vitamin B6, and vitamin B12, can send your mood on a downhill slide. Look for a multivitamin/mineral supplement that contains at least 100 percent of the recommended dietary allowance for these nutrients.

❖ **Anticipate the action and your reaction.** You'll often find coping with major life changes easier if you try to anticipate and be prepared for these events.

If nothing lifts the gloom that seems to surround you, see your doctor. If you feel suicidal, talk to someone immediately. No one to confide in? Check your phone book for a local suicide hot line or mental health crisis number, or seek help at the emergency room. But don't give up. Researchers have made major strides in antidepressant therapy in the past few years. It may only take a few weeks until you're feeling better.

A SAD story

For many, winter is a time of jolliness and good cheer. But if you feel more like the grumpy old grinch than jolly old St. Nick, you may be suffering from seasonal affective disorder (SAD).

Since low light is the most common trigger of SAD, the disorder occurs more often during the winter. However, this doesn't mean you have to feel sad during those times. Follow these tips for a lighter, brighter mood all year long.

❖ Get more light. Weather permitting, get out of the house and walk as often as possible. Flood your house with sunshine. Pull up the blinds, push back the curtains. Turn on all the lights in the room.

❖ Get up at the crack of dawn. For whatever reason, early morning light makes many SAD sufferers feel much better.

❖ Watch what you eat. Distract yourself from overeating by involving yourself in other activities you enjoy. Be especially careful not to buy or store extra sweets and starches in your house.

❖ Treat yourself to a winter vacation in some warm sunny spot.

❖ Learn stress management techniques. Meditation is a good option. Start with a five-minute session and gradually work up to 20 minutes. Mental relaxation helps reduce stress.

❖ Contact the SAD sufferers support group NOSAD at P.O. Box 40133, Washington, D.C. 20016.

If self-help doesn't clear up your SAD, see your doctor. He may prescribe antidepressants or light therapy.

Diarrhea

Frequent, watery discharge of stool

It's been referred to as Montezuma's revenge. That unpleasant rumbling in your gut followed by a mad dash for the nearest restroom. Occasional diarrhea is a common problem, usually caused by bacteria or a virus.

Travelers often get diarrhea when they ask their digestive systems to cope with strange food and water. One flight attendant even discovered that her seemingly innocent sugar-free gum was the source of her severe diarrhea. When she sought medical help, she found that her gum contained sorbitol, a sugar substitute, which acts as a laxative because the body can't digest it. Before you swear off sugar-free gum, however, you should know that this woman chewed up to 60 sticks every day.

Fortunately, most bouts of diarrhea are temporary, and your body deals with it. However, if your diarrhea is severe or continues for a long time, you may become dangerously dehydrated, so see your doctor.

It's time to see your doctor if you have diarrhea and:

- Fever
- Abdominal pain spasms
- Unexplained weight loss

If your battles with diarrhea seem to come and go, and you also have the above symptoms, you may have Crohn's disease. No one knows what causes this chronic disease, but more people seem to be affected by it every day.

- Excessive weight loss
- Nausea and vomiting

- Gas and bloating
- Rectal itching

If you have these symptoms, you may have an intestinal parasite. The thought of worms may be unpleasant, but it can happen to the best of us.

- Fatigue
- Unexplained weight loss
- Vomiting
- Abdominal pain

These are the symptoms of a rare disorder called celiac sprue disease. This disease causes gluten to damage the lining of your small intestine. Gluten is a protein found in wheat, barley, and rye, and the only treatment is to avoid all foods that have it. Rice, corn, and soybean flour are good substitutes. The only way to diagnose the disease is to see your doctor.

- Vomiting
- Stomach pain
- Diarrhea (sometimes bloody)
- Other people who ate the same food as you also get sick

If you have these symptoms after eating a meal, you may have a form of food poisoning. Depending on the type of poison, you may feel sick as early as one hour after eating contaminated food or as long as three to five days after. Though most cases of food poisoning will run their course without serious complications, severe cases should be treated by a doctor. (See also *Abdominal pain, sudden* chapter.)

- Nausea and vomiting
- Stomach pain
- Flushed or pale skin
- Itching
- Respiratory distress (coughing, wheezing, breathlessness)

This may indicate a food allergy. Keeping a food diary will help you identify potential culprits, and eliminating those foods may be the only treatment you need. However, a serious allergic reaction, known as anaphylaxis, can be fatal. If you have breathing difficulty or pass out, you need immediate help.

- Nausea
- Loss of appetite (which may lead to weight loss)
- Cramping abdominal pain that is usually relieved by bowel movements
- It alternates with constipation

Irritable bowel syndrome (IBS) is usually just an annoyance and does not cause any serious damage. But if it interferes with your lifestyle by keeping you away from public functions, discuss it with your doctor.

Immediate help for IBS

Irritable bowel syndrome may not be a life-threatening condition, but it can certainly make you irritable. Your colon (large intestine) is supposed to squeeze slowly and steadily to move waste material toward your rectum. Occasionally, stronger contractions result in a bowel movement. If you have irritable bowel syndrome, however, your colon has no self-control. It may squeeze too hard, rushing food through your system quickly, resulting in cramps and diarrhea. Or it may not squeeze hard enough, so food sits in your body too long, making you feel bloated and constipated. Some people may experience alternating periods of diarrhea and constipation with IBS.

Doctors don't know for sure what causes IBS, but stress and diet are the most likely answers. Eating normally triggers contractions of your colon, which often leads to a bowel movement 30 to 60 minutes after a meal. Many people with IBS, however, may have cramps and diarrhea much sooner after a meal. The strength of those contractions may depend on what and how much you eat. Fat in particular seems to set off strong colon contractions. Stress may also trigger colon contractions in people with IBS.

When you are suffering the ups and downs of irritable bowel syndrome, you may be tempted to reach for an over-the-counter laxative or other medicines for a quick fix. However, you could end up depending on laxatives, which would weaken your intestines in the long run. See your doctor if IBS interferes with your life. He may prescribe fiber supplements or tranquilizers to help you relax. But self help may be the most sensible, long-lasting solution to IBS.

The long-range plan for IBS

If you have irritable bowel syndrome, the bad news is that you'll probably have to deal with it for years to come. The good news is it doesn't cause permanent damage to your digestive system, and it doesn't lead to more serious problems. It is also controllable. Try some of these hints to soothe and calm that cranky bowel.

- ❖ **Add fiber to your diet.** A high-fiber diet may make your colon's job easier and lessen the chances of colon spasms. When it comes to IBS, however, all fiber is not created equal. Some forms of fiber may actually make IBS symptoms worse. Some people find that certain citrus fruits and bran give them a problem. Try whole-grain products and high-fiber fruits and vegetables. Products that contain psyllium, like Fiberall and Metamucil, may be helpful.
- ❖ **Learn what foods make your IBS worse.** You may need to steer clear of certain foods. Although food triggers may be different for each person, the more common culprits include fatty fried foods, and spicy or sugary foods. If lactose intolerance is contributing to your IBS, you need to limit the dairy products you eat.
- ❖ **Cut the caffeine.** Caffeine may stimulate you and keep you awake, but it may also stimulate your colon, causing diarrhea.
- ❖ **Eat small.** Large meals can set off cramps and diarrhea in people with IBS. You may want to try to eat smaller, more frequent meals to avoid these problems.

105

- ❖ **Exercise.** Believe it or not, your bowels work better when you exercise regularly. Exercise is also relaxing, and since stress contributes to IBS, moving your body may ease your IBS in more ways than one.
- ❖ **Lower your stress.** Although this is obviously easier said than done, lowering your stress level may help relieve the pain in your gut. Take time out of your busy day to listen to soothing music, read a relaxing novel, or take a brisk walk. If you have a huge amount of stress in your life, counseling may help.

Dizziness

A feeling of unsteadiness on your feet
A sensation that the room is spinning violently and
*   you are about to fall*

Simple things can cause temporary dizziness. When you stand up suddenly and feel dizzy, it's probably just a harmless drop in your blood pressure. If riding in a boat or airplane causes dizziness, it's probably motion sickness. And if you're worried or frightened when the sensation hits you, the dizziness could be from a bad case of anxiety or even a panic attack.

If you feel dizzy soon after you've taken a new medicine, whether it's over-the-counter or by prescription, you may be having a drug reaction. Don't take it again, and call your doctor. Here are some other situations in which you should get your doctor's help.

 It's time to see your doctor if you have dizziness and:

- Daily severe headaches
- Drowsiness

- Confusion
- Paralysis on one side of your body

If these symptoms follow a head injury, see your doctor immediately. You might have a hemorrhage, or bleeding, in your brain.

- Exposure to hot weather
- Faintness and weakness
- Cramps in your muscles
- Rapid or extremely slow heartbeat

These are the signals of heatstroke or heat exhaustion. Too much heat has built up in your body, and it is not able to cool down. This is a medical emergency, so get help immediately. (See also *Muscle cramps or weakness* chapter.)

- Faintness and weakness
- Breathing difficulty
- Tiredness
- Irregular heartbeat that feels like a fluttering in your chest

You may have atrial fibrillation, in which your heart beats irregularly and too fast. Your heart may feel as if it's flopping around in your chest. This type of irregular heartbeat may resolve itself, but it is usually dangerous if left untreated, so you need to see your doctor.

- Extremely slow heartbeat (60 or fewer beats per minute)
- Sudden weakness or fatigue

These are the symptoms of bradycardia, or slow heartbeat. With this condition, your heart may slow down too much and just stop beating. Bradycardia is normal in a well-conditioned athlete, but not in most other people. You may have an underlying disease, or your heart medicine, such as a beta-blocker, is slowing your heart rate too much.

- Nausea or vomiting
- Loss of vision or visual disturbances

Cure that after-dinner dizziness

There's a good reason for lingering after a meal with a steaming cup of coffee or tea. More than just a pleasant ritual, the cup of brew may keep you from an unpleasant bout of dizziness.

Most people's blood pressure drops immediately after a meal. The name for this is postprandial (after-meal) hypotension (low blood pressure). It can make you lightheaded and dizzy when you try to stand up, and even cause you to faint. You may have these symptoms even if you normally have high blood pressure.

The caffeine in a cup of coffee or tea can raise your blood pressure just enough to prevent the dizziness and faintness. Getting up and walking around also will raise your blood pressure enough to prevent the symptoms, but it's best to wait until you feel stable on your feet. A little caffeine will safely do the trick.

So savor your after-dinner coffee or tea to keep yourself in perfect balance. Maybe you'll enjoy some fascinating after-dinner conversation as well.

- **Seizures**
- **Severe headache**

You may have a brain tumor. See your doctor immediately for a checkup.

- **Faintness**
- **Recurring headache**
- **Nausea and vomiting**
- **Breathing problems**

These symptoms signal carbon monoxide poisoning, usually from some kind of heating system, engine, or industrial fumes. You must find the source of the carbon monoxide and fix it. Carbon monoxide poisoning can cause death. (See also *Headache* chapter.)

108

- Headache
- Blurred vision or double vision
- Weakness in your arms or legs
- Slurred speech

You may be having a transient ischemic attack (TIA), which is a temporary brain disturbance that usually clears up within 24 hours. It's also possible you have had a mild stroke. See your doctor immediately. (See also *Slurred speech* chapter.)

- Headache
- Confusion
- Blurred vision
- Vomiting

If you have recently lost consciousness following a head injury, and experience these symptoms along with dizziness, you may have a concussion.

- A stiff neck
- Pain in your neck that extends to your shoulders and arms
- Weakness and loss of sensation in your fingers, hands, and arms

These symptoms point to cervical spondylosis, a pressure on the nerves in your neck caused by arthritis or bone deterioration.

- Ear noise and hearing loss
- Uncontrolled eye movement
- Nausea and vomiting

If these symptoms accompany severe attacks of dizziness, they point to labyrinthitis or Meniere's disease, both serious disorders of the inner ear. If your hearing is okay and it happens only when you move your head, it may be benign paroxysmal positional vertigo, a temporary disorder.

The long-range plan for vertigo

You wake up in the middle of the night and sense that something is wrong. As you turn to your right side, you know, even in the dark, that the room is spinning wildly around you. You haven't been transported to a scene from a Hitchcock movie; you're a victim of vertigo.

One of the most common diseases of the inner ear is benign paroxysmal positional vertigo, or BPPV. It affects 15 to 40 percent of people who go to doctors for help with their dizziness. BPPV usually occurs for the first time between the ages of 30 and 50, and it's twice as likely to strike you if you're a woman.

When you have BPPV, it's hard to concentrate on anything else. You just want an end to the horrible spinning sensation and nausea you get every time you turn your head the wrong way or try to lie down or stand up. But if your doctor diagnoses your dizziness as benign paroxysmal positional vertigo, you're lucky. First, your ailment has a definite name and cause, and second, there's something your doctor can do about it.

A tiny, complex system within your inner ear keeps your body in balance most of the time. BPPV occurs when calcium particles inside the mechanism float around or are knocked out of place and into the wrong position. When you move your head a certain way, it sends the wrong signals to your brain. This miscommunication results in vertigo, the feeling that the room is spinning violently around you. Nausea and sometimes vomiting are also part of the sensation. A blow to the head or a viral infection may cause BPPV, but usually you don't know why it comes on.

If you do nothing and just live with the misery, BPPV should go away within a few months. But there's no reason why you shouldn't get help and get over it. When you go to your doctor, he'll give you a test called the Hallpike maneuver to check for the condition. At this point, he'll be watching your eye movements to help in his diagnosis. Now comes the surprising part.

If his medical knowledge is up-to-date, your doctor can perform a five-minute procedure called the Epley maneuver, named after the doctor who invented it. He'll have you lie on the examining table with your head hanging off the end and turned toward the "bad" side. Then he'll rotate your head 180 degrees. The turning action should pop the calcium particles out of their hiding place and back into the right location. The Semont maneuver is another process your doctor might use to reposition the "ear rocks."

At home, you need to keep your head upright for 48 hours, even when you sleep. A recliner chair or a sofa with fluffy pillows can help you sleep comfortably and at the correct angle. For at least a week, be extra careful in the way you move your head. Sleep on two pillows, don't sleep on the "bad" side, and don't do any exercises that move your head quickly, such as sit-ups or toe touches. Also, don't go to the hairdresser or dentist, or bend your head while you shave or wash your hair.

Once your doctor has shown you the correct way to do the Epley maneuver, you can try it on your own if you have another run-in with BPPV. You must do it correctly, though, or you may lodge the calcium particles more firmly in the wrong place and prolong your vertigo.

Don't live with dizziness if it seems the cause is as simple as BPPV. Get your doctor's help. If your regular doctor doesn't know the Epley maneuver, find one who does. An otolaryngologist, or "ear, nose, and throat" doctor should be able to help you stop the spinning.

Drowsiness

Feeling sleepy or half-asleep
Sluggishness that interferes with your daily activities

Many things in life influence your sleep patterns and energy levels. Stress, anxiety, and depression are mental states that can keep you up at night and down during the day. Activities such as shift work, excessive drinking, or traveling will throw off your internal sleep clock. And viruses, allergies, and illnesses are treats from Mother Nature that can leave you tired and sluggish. If you have that slow, lazy feeling a little too often, or regularly find yourself fighting to keep your eyes open, examine your routine and try to determine the cause.

Is alcohol part of your lunch menu, or have you recently cut out caffeine? Either one of these will lower your energy and make you feel sleepy. Are you skipping breakfast, eating a heavy dinner, or snacking on high-sugar foods? Are you sitting around the house too much, getting too little sleep at night, or maybe even too much? These are all easy to fix once you recognize the problem. However, if you have eliminated routine causes and still find yourself dangerously drowsy during the day, you could have a more serious problem, calling for more serious action.

It's time to see your doctor if you have drowsiness and:

Recently received a blow to the head

You may be suffering from a blood clot or swelling under the skull.

Headaches
Blurred vision
Weakness in your arms or legs
Difficulty speaking
Dizziness

It is possible you had a mild stroke. See your doctor immediately. (See also *Slurred speech* chapter.)

Boredom, fatigue
Changes in eating habits
Loss of interest in sex
Feelings of guilt or anxiety
Various pains without obvious cause
Thoughts of death
Mood swings and bad temper

Don't dismiss any of these symptoms as trivial. You could be suffering from depression, a very real and crippling illness. Treatment is available, however, so get help. (See also *Depression* chapter.)

112

- Frequent periods of sudden sleep
- Attacks of waking paralysis set off by strong emotions
- Intense dreams just after falling asleep or just before waking
- Brief, sudden loss of muscle control, sometimes causing collapse
- Lapse of recent memory, even in the middle of an activity
- Frequent nighttime awakenings
- Blurred vision

Narcolepsy is a rare sleeping disorder that can easily be misdiagnosed, but dream-like hallucinations and paralysis help to identify this condition. If you are diagnosed with narcolepsy, protect yourself from those sudden sleep attacks by not driving long distances or working with dangerous machinery.

Take medication

Tranquilizers, sleeping pills, antihistamines in cough and cold medicines, heart pills, and allergy remedies all have elements in them that will cause drowsiness. Check with your doctor for possible side effects of any medication you are on.

- Loud, long, and frequent snoring
- Weight problems
- Early morning headaches
- Nighttime breathing difficulties
- Sexual dysfunction

These symptoms indicate you may suffer from sleep apnea. Because it makes you so drowsy during the day, many experts believe it causes thousands of accidents on the road and in the workplace.

Immediate help for sleep apnea

If the air flow through your nose or mouth is blocked, or your brain sends out the wrong cues, you may stop breathing while you sleep. Your body reacts to the lack of oxygen by triggering a gasping reflex, waking you enough to start your breathing again. Victims of sleep apnea usually suffer at least 30 of these episodes during the night, each lasting 10 seconds or longer.

Millions of Americans suffer from sleep apnea, but it affects middle-aged men twice as much as women. People with large necks are more likely to have the condition because they usually have some type of blockage in the nose or back of the throat. Tobacco, alcohol or sleeping pills will make the condition worse. If you suffer from sleep apnea, you are more likely to have high blood pressure, heart attack, and stroke. The condition also seems to run in families.

You may suffer from sleep apnea and not know it. Examine the list of symptoms, and have your spouse keep a watchful eye on you at night. What might seem like simple snoring could be a gasp for life.

* ❖ **Try not to sleep on your back.** Sew a tennis or ping pong ball into a pocket on the back of your pajamas. The discomfort will make you sleep on your side.

* ❖ **Skip that after-dinner cocktail.** Alcohol will play havoc with your sleep patterns. While it may at first seem to make you sleepier, the overall quality of sleep is poor. Instead try a soothing, decaffeinated hot drink before bedtime.

* ❖ **Reduce stress.** By lowering your anxiety or depression, you improve your chances for a deeper sleep. Thinking about your problems before you fall asleep will only anchor the tension in your subconscious. Try some gentle stretching and deep-breathing exercises before bedtime, focusing on a routine that will calm and relax you.

The long-range plan for sleep apnea

Once your doctor has diagnosed your condition, he can judge whether it calls for drastic measures.

* ❖ **Lose weight.** Statistics show that sleep apnea is more common if you're overweight. A safe, gradual weight-loss program, supervised by a doctor, will make you healthier and improve the quality of

your sleep. Avoid vigorous exercise just before bedtime, however. By saving these activities for morning or early evening, you allow your body to wind down and prepare for sleep.

❖ **Guard your mouth.** A properly fitted mouth guard, worn while sleeping, can reposition your jaw and tongue so your throat stays open.

❖ **Mask it.** A new treatment for sleep apnea forces your airway to stay open by blowing air from a compressor into a face mask you wear over your nose and mouth.

❖ **Seek surgery.** Doctors can shift your jaw forward, remove any tissue in the back of your throat, and attach a pacemaker to stimulate your diaphragm and help your breathing. This is probably the only course that will cure sleep apnea.

It is common for older men and women to experience daytime sleepiness, and a brief rest to recharge your batteries is not a bad idea. If you lead an active social life, are in reasonably good health, and not overweight, that power nap should only enhance your life, not diminish it. So whenever you feel those doldrums, go ahead and take a siesta. You'll feel fresh and alert again in no time.

Ear problems

Pain in your ears
Noise inside your ears
Hearing loss

Your ears house one of the most delicate and complex systems in your body. Through an almost magical process, sound waves are captured, carried, and converted into impulses that your brain interprets as sound. Tiny bones, microscopic haircells, and thin membranes accomplish the enormous task of bringing you music, laughter and poetry. But because this system is so complex, an overwhelming number of things can go wrong.

As you age, you lose nerve cells that you can't replace, and vital parts of your ear begin to break down. Age-related hearing loss affects nearly one-fourth of the population over 65. If you count yourself among them, don't despair. You have hundreds of aids to help improve your hearing and your quality of life. Remember, using a hearing aid is not a sign of weakness, but rather a declaration of strength.

Problems such as pain, noise, or mild hearing loss can affect your balance, your mood, and your daily activities. Don't put off seeing a doctor since these signs could indicate a more serious problem.

It's time to see your doctor if you have:

- Ear noise
- Hearing loss
- Dizziness
- Uncontrolled eye movement
- Nausea and vomiting

These symptoms could point to labyrinthitis or Meniere's disease, both serious disorders of the inner ear.

- Ear pain
- A stuffy nose with a green-yellow discharge
- Tension, fullness or pressure in the face and head
- Throbbing headache made worse by bending over
- Pain behind the eyes and behind the cheeks that feels like a toothache
- Loss of sense of smell
- Fever, chills, cough, or sore throat

Your sinuses are air-filled pockets and passageways in the bones around your nose that connect your nose, eyes, and ears. When your sinuses become irritated and inflamed by allergies, pollution, smoke, or a viral infection, you can develop sinusitis. (See also *Nose, runny or stuffy* chapter.)

- Sudden intense ear pain
- Hearing loss
- Ringing in your ear
- Plugged feeling in your ear
- Fever
- Discharge from your ear

Otitis media is the medical term for a middle ear infection. It occurs when a bacterium or virus spreads to the middle ear by way of the eustachian tube (the slender passage that connects the middle ear and the back of the throat). This most often happens when you have a cold or the flu. However, allergies and sinusitis can also cause a middle ear infection.

- Itching in and around your ear
- Ear pain made worse when your earlobe is pulled
- Partial hearing loss
- Redness and swelling in the ear canal
- Discharge from your ear
- Slight fever

These symptoms indicate an infection in the outer ear canal called otitis externa or swimmers' ear. It is caused by bacteria that settle on the skin in and around the ear canal, and usually means you have too much moisture in your ears.

- Slow hearing loss
- Ringing in your ears
- Dizziness
- Better hearing in noisy surroundings

Otosclerosis is a hereditary condition in which a growth forms in the middle ear. This prevents one of the small bones from vibrating and passing sound waves on to the inner ear. Your doctor may recommend a hearing aid or surgery.

- Ear pain
- Fever
- Ache or throbbing pain in a tooth
- Pain when chewing or biting

- Swollen, red and sore gum around tooth
- Swollen and tender glands in neck and side of face
- Bad-tasting discharge in mouth

Bacteria sometimes reach the nerves and blood vessels inside a tooth, or the area between the teeth and gums, causing an infection. If this infection spreads into the tissue and bone surrounding the tooth, an abscess develops. See your dentist as soon as possible.

- Ringing, roaring, or buzzing sound in your ears
- Some hearing loss
- Feeling of pressure in your ears
- A muscle ache in front of your ears, from your temples to your neck
- Clicking, cracking or crunching noises when moving your jaw
- Difficulty opening your mouth completely or moving your jaw from side to side
- Dizziness or nausea

If you suffer from a mix of these symptoms, chances are you have been diagnosed with anything from a toothache or a migraine to a sinus infection. But, like 20 million other Americans, you may have a completely legitimate condition called temporomandibular joint syndrome or TMJ. (See also *Jaw pain* chapter.)

- Sudden ear pain
- Partial hearing loss
- Ringing in your ear
- Dizziness
- Bleeding or discharge from your ear
- Recent ear or head injury
- Recent middle ear infection

Sharp objects inserted into the ear, sudden air pressure changes, or a severe ear infection can all cause your eardrum to rupture or burst. This leaves the tiny bones of the middle ear exposed to damage or infection, which can lead to hearing loss. With a doctor's care, your eardrum should heal in about two months.

- Ear pain
- Sneezing
- Fatigue
- Runny or stuffy nose
- Itchy, watery eyes
- Itchy nose and scratchy throat

These are the symptoms of allergic rhinitis, commonly known as an "allergy." It's usually caused by your body's reaction to pollen, dust mites, mold, or animals.

- Ear pain
- Headache
- Cough
- Sore throat
- Low-grade fever
- Fatigue
- Runny nose and watery eyes

If you are suffering from these symptoms, you probably have the most common illness in the world — a cold. Like the flu, a cold is caused by a virus (any one of 200 or so, at last count), but it's a less serious illness than influenza. (See also *Nose, runny or stuffy* chapter.)

- Hearing loss
- Ringing in your ears
- Medication

Several drugs can damage the inner ear. Check with your doctor if you experience some hearing loss while taking streptomycin, erythromycin, gentamicin, quinine, furosemide, ethacrynic acid, bumetanide or heavy doses of aspirin. More than 200 prescription and non-prescription drugs advise that ear ringing is a possible side effect.

- Ear pain
- Some loss of hearing
- Plugged feeling in your ear
- Ringing in your ear

Sometimes, the glands in your ear canal produce too much wax, blocking the canal and affecting your hearing. You can buy special drops that will soften and help remove this buildup. If you don't feel comfortable removing the earwax yourself, or if you have a ruptured eardrum, see your doctor.

- Ear pain
- Feeling of tension in your eardrum
- Partial hearing loss
- Dizziness
- Ringing in your ear
- Recent travel, usually by plane

Changes in air pressure sometimes cause painful stress in your ears. If you have a cold or an ear infection and must travel, see your pharmacist for a decongestant. If you have completed your travel but still have the symptoms, you may have damaged your middle ear. Your doctor can prescribe a strong prescription decongestant, a steroid nasal spray, or antibiotics.

- Buzzing noises in your ear
- Intense tickling feeling in your ear

These symptoms could mean you have an insect trapped in your ear canal. You can gently float it out by filling the canal with water, or see your doctor.

- Noises inside your ear, such as a ring, buzz, roar, whistle, hiss, chirp, squeal, or whine, when there is no outer sound present
- Partial hearing loss

Tinnitus, or "head noises" as it is sometimes called, is a symptom of many different conditions and is often a result of other disorders, yet it can occur on its own as well.

Immediate help for tinnitus

Millions of people suffer from tinnitus. For some, it is no more than an occasional annoyance. Others experience continual noise that causes overwhelming stress.

Because tinnitus can be a by-product of so many other conditions, it is possible that by discovering and treating another disorder, your tinnitus will go away. Besides the conditions listed earlier in this chapter, some of the possible causes are high or low blood pressure, a tumor, diabetes, thyroid problems, a head or neck aneurysm, syphilis, atherosclerosis, or anemia. See a specialist in this area, an otolaryngologist or otologist, to rule out any treatable condition. If you come away with a clean bill of health, but are still hearing noises in your ears, don't think you are crazy. It is possible to have tinnitus by itself. While there is no cure, experts say you can learn to cope with the condition.

❖ **Cut the clamor.** Studies show a connection between long-range exposure to loud noises and tinnitus. If your job involves loud music or machinery, or you spend lots of time around sporting events, motors, or tools, you may gradually feel the effects of tinnitus. To conserve your hearing, you should try to avoid the noise if you can. If that's not possible, then use ear plugs or muffs, spend as little time as possible in the noisy environment, and try to lower the sound.

❖ **Put down the pick-me-up.** The mechanisms in your ear rely heavily on the nervous system to make it work. If you overstimulate your nerves, you could make your tinnitus worse. Try to avoid stimulants like nicotine, alcohol, and caffeine.

❖ **Sounds to sleep by.** Many tinnitus sufferers find they can't fall asleep because of all the noise in their ears. So, relax, wind down, get comfortable, and maybe put on some soothing music. Relaxation tapes and environmental sounds can help block the noise, too. If you prefer, you can turn on a fan, tune in to static on the radio, or put the TV on low.

The long-range plan for tinnitus

Learning to live with tinnitus may be the greatest challenge you will ever face.

❖ **Call time out.** Anyone who suffers from tinnitus knows just how stressful the constant noise can be. Unfortunately, anxiety will only make your condition worse. If you can learn to control your emotional response, you can break the cycle. There are many stress-reducing techniques available; you just need to find what works best for you. Some easy steps to begin with are deep breathing, tension-releasing exercises, and mental imagery.

❖ **Get physical.** Exercising every day will not only improve your overall health, but your mental health as well. Find an activity you enjoy, and stick with it. You will feel stronger, and it may distract you from your discomfort. You may even find it's a good way to take out your frustrations with your condition.

❖ **Stay positive.** Tinnitus may very well be a permanent part of your life, but that doesn't mean it has to defeat you. Keep trying different treatments until you find the one that works for you.

❖ **Learn how to help yourself.** Biofeedback is a technique where you learn to control otherwise automatic functions of your body, like heart rate and blood pressure. This, in turn, will allow you to control your stress. Hypnosis and acupuncture have not been proven successful in every case, but under a professional's care, you might find they work for you.

❖ **Education is hope.** Learn about your condition. Tinnitus can be frightening, but rest assured it is not life threatening, nor a sign of mental illness or stroke. The condition also does not cause deafness, although you may experience some hearing loss.

❖ **Seek support.** Join a tinnitus self-help group like the American Tinnitus Association (ATA), get professional counseling, and don't be afraid to talk about it with your family and friends. They need to understand your condition, too.

If you need more intensive treatment to cope with your tinnitus, you may want to consider one of these:

❖ Hearing aids can increase the sound level around you, making it easier to ignore the sounds you hear in your head. A hearing aid also will help with any hearing loss you may have.

❖ Tinnitus maskers look like hearing aids, but they make a specific noise designed to cover the type of tinnitus sound you hear.

❖ A tinnitus instrument combines the functions of both a hearing aid and a masker.

Eye problems

Itchy, watery, red, painful, or dry, scratchy eyes

Your eyes are your most important tool for experiencing the world around you. They're your windows to a golden sunrise, a velvet pink rose, or a baby's first smile. When your eyes itch, burn, or hurt, they affect your whole attitude.

Some eye problems have simple solutions that you can fix yourself. If a cold makes your eyes itchy and watery, an over-the-counter cold medicine may help. If your eyes are dry, you can buy artificial tears to supplement your own. But some problems are more complicated, and your doctor needs to check them out.

 ## It's time to see your doctor if you have:

- Severe eye pain
- Redness in your eye
- Tenderness, swelling, or bleeding in your eye
- Blurred vision

These symptoms could indicate an injury, inflammation, infection, or ulcer of your eye (corneal ulcer) or something lodged in your eye. All these situations are medical emergencies; you need to see your doctor immediately.

- A sudden episode of seeing spots and flashes of light
- Blurred vision
- Gradual dimming or loss of your vision

These are the symptoms of a detached retina, a tearing or separation of your retina from the rest of your eye. The retina is the part of your eye that enables you to see light. You don't feel pain when your retina detaches, but you may suddenly lose your vision. Get to a doctor immediately. The sooner a surgeon can reattach your retina, the better chance you have of regaining your sight.

- Headache
- Fever
- Neck stiffness
- Nausea and vomiting
- Eyes that are sensitive to bright light

If you have these symptoms, you might have meningitis, which is an infection of the spinal fluid and the tissues around the brain and spinal cord.

- Pain and redness in your eye
- A gritty or itchy feeling in your eye
- A swollen, painful, or red eyelid
- An eyelid turned inward or outward
- A lump on your eyelid that doesn't go away in a few days
- A drooping eyelid

Problems with your eyelids may turn out to be minor, but you should see your doctor to make sure they stay that way. The problem could be an infection such as blepharitis or conjunctivitis, also known as pinkeye. A lump on your eyelid could be a simple sty or chalazion, the inflammation of a gland that lubricates your eyelid. A drooping upper eyelid, called ptosis, could indicate an underlying disease.

- Bulging eyes
- Blurred or double vision

A common cause of bulging eyes is an overactive thyroid gland. Bulging eyes can also mean something more serious, such as an infection, blood clot, or tumor behind your eye. See your doctor to find out. (See also *Weight changes, unexplained* chapter.)

- Constant dryness of your eyes, mouth, and nose
- Vaginal dryness that makes intercourse painful
- Painful, achy joints

Dry eyes can mean your body's tear production is simply slowing down with age and not producing as much lubrication for your eyes as it used to. But combined with these other symptoms, constant dry eyes can point to Sjogren's syndrome, an autoimmune disorder. (See also *Mouth dryness* chapter.)

- Red, teary eye
- Blurred vision
- An enlarged pupil

If you also have a throbbing headache pain around your eye, you could have glaucoma.

- Itchy, watery eyes
- Scratchy throat
- Sneezing
- Fatigue
- Runny or stuffy nose
- Dark circles under your eyes

These are the symptoms of allergic rhinitis, commonly known as allergy or hay fever. It's usually caused by your body's reaction to pollen, dust mites, mold, or animals, but it can be a reaction to certain foods, chemicals, or environmental pollutants.

Immediate help for allergy

When you're suffering through the itchy eyes, runny nose, sneezing, and general discomfort of an allergy attack, don't blame your body — it's just doing its job. These symptoms are actually a sign that your immune system is protecting you by fighting off invaders. But these substances aren't life-threatening bacteria or viruses; they're ordinary things like grass pollen, dust, animal dander, or mold spores.

Your immune system makes antibodies to defend you against foreign substances — in this case, allergens — that invade your body. To fight the invaders, your antibodies send out chemicals such as histamines, which, unfortunately, irritate and inflame your tissues. A lot of this activity takes place in your eyes, nose, lungs, stomach, and intestines, which is why you end up with itchy eyes, sneezing, runny nose, and sometimes, vomiting and diarrhea. When you're feeling miserable from these constant battles, here are some tips that can help.

❖ **Find the culprit.** The first step in fighting your allergy is to figure out what is causing it. If you have a sneezing fit every time you get near a cat, chances are the cat's the problem. If your eyes itch and your nose runs when you walk into a certain room, you may be allergic to dust mites, microscopic animals that thrive in dust. Sneezing and sniffling in the spring and fall probably means seasonal allergies, known as hay fever. Your doctor can help you figure out which allergen is bothering you. An allergy skin test or a blood test can usually pinpoint just what's causing your misery.

❖ **Get some relief.** If you reach the point where you just can't stand the sneezing and itching, you may need to turn to medication. An over-the-counter antihistamine will knock out those bothersome histamines, but it may knock you out as well. If so, get a prescription for one that won't make you drowsy. Decongestants can help relieve your stuffy nose, but if you get a nasal spray, you shouldn't use it for more than three days at a time. Saline spray can safely relieve a dry, itchy nose.

For hay fever, prescription steroid nasal sprays work wonders. Ask your doctor about trying them. If your allergies come back every year,

126

you may want to consider immunotherapy, a method in which you gradually get desensitized to the allergens that bother you. It is a series of shots given over several allergy seasons. After two or three seasons, you may be able to live more comfortably with your allergy.

❖ **Have a cup of joe.** If you have hay fever, drinking more coffee may help you breathe easier. A California study of people with hay fever found that taking caffeine helped relieve allergy symptoms. Just be sure to weigh the side effects of coffee against the good effects if you decide to go for that extra cup.

❖ **Try some vitamin C.** You heard it could cure the common cold. Now some doctors believe it may be the best treatment for seasonal allergies. Even if you already take a vitamin C supplement, you might want to increase your dosage and see if it helps. Doctors recommend taking 500 milligrams (mg) up to 4 grams (about a teaspoon) a day. Try it in a powdered form mixed into fruit juice or a carbonated drink. But if you take large doses of vitamin C, only do so for a week or two when your allergy is at its worst. And if you have high blood pressure or kidney problems, look for vitamin C without sodium ascorbate, a form of salt.

❖ **Get help from honey.** Another treatment for seasonal allergies may be as near as your neighborhood grocery store. Honey made in local hives contains traces of pollen from surrounding plants. If you regularly eat local honey, you're desensitizing yourself to seasonal allergens the same way that immunotherapy does. You need to take one to three teaspoons of honey a day for an extended time (no one knows exactly how long) to get the sweet benefits.

❖ **Watch the wine.** If you tend to have allergies or sinus problems, it's probably a good idea to stay away from red wine. Red wine makes your blood vessels expand, causing sinus pressure. That, in turn, causes fatigue and other allergy symptoms.

If you want to drink wine, stick to white or blush instead.

❖ **Pick your pets.** If you're considering a pet, skip the fluff and fur. Pet dander and fleas are common allergens for allergy-prone people. Your best pet bets are fish, turtles, frogs, lizards, and sand crabs.

❖ **Care for kitty or pooch.** If you're one of the millions of people who already own a dog, cat, or other furry of fluffy pet, you need to take extra care to keep your pet from contributing to your allergies. Here are some things you can do:

- Keep your pet outside. A fenced yard, along with a sturdy house or a warm garage, should be plenty of shelter for your animal companion, especially if he makes you sneeze and sniffle when he stays inside.

- Get your pet treated for fleas. It may actually be the fleas you're allergic to instead of the dog or cat. Your vet has effective flea treatments available.

- Bathe your pet often, or have someone else do it. This will cut down on the amount of hair and dander that float around in the air, ready to cause your allergy symptoms.

- Change the filter in your home's cooling or heating system often. Also consider putting filters inside your heating and cooling vents to trap more allergy-causing pet particles before they blow back into the rooms of your house.

❖ **Close those windows.** Spring and fall are the best times to ride in your car with the top off, the sunroof open, or the windows down. These are also the worst times of year for allergy sufferers. Riding in an open car simply exposes you to more allergens, and the blowing air forces more of them into your eyes, nose, and throat.

At home, you may be tempted by beautiful weather to fling your windows wide open to enjoy the fresh air. The breeze may feel wonderful, but you'll pay a price with more sneezing and sniffling.

Let the heating and cooling systems in your car and home do some of the dirty work for you and filter out the dust, pollen, and other outside allergens that make you suffer. Enjoy the beautiful spring and fall weather with your windows closed, and you'll greet it with a smile instead of tears.

❖ **Protect yourself in the yard.** If you can, invest in a professional dust mask — the kind carpenters use in their workshops. If you can't find one, go to your local discount store and get a package of disposable filter masks you can wear whenever you do a job that exposes you to pollen, mold, or dust. They're inexpensive, and they're good insurance for keeping your gardening and grass cutting chores from becoming an introduction to allergy misery. A pair of sunglasses, especially the kind that wrap around your eye area, will do a good job of protecting your eyes from allergens. The best time to schedule outside chores is probably mid-morning. In the early evening, pollen is worse as it's settling to the ground.

❖ **Wash up.** If you've been working in the garden or just spending time outside, your clothes are likely to be full of pollen and dust. Take them off and wash them when you come inside, and you'll get rid of a big source of allergens. Your hair acts as a magnet for pollen and dust, so wash it before you go to bed to get a more comfortable night's sleep.

The long-range plan for allergy

The best plan for dealing with allergic rhinitis in the long run is, of course, to avoid the things in your life that cause it. But that isn't always possible. The next best plan is to do what you can to protect yourself from allergy as much as possible. Here are some tips to try:

❖ **Supplement with C.** New evidence says that taking vitamin C on a long-term basis can lower the amount of histamine in your blood. Remember, histamine is the chemical that causes an allergic response in your eyes and nose, so if you have less in your body, you'll have fewer symptoms. Since vitamin C acts as a natural antihistamine, you may be able to cut down on the drugs you take for your allergy. A supplement of 500 mg a day should be plenty to give you the full benefits of vitamin C. But you should also aim to get most of your vitamin C from food, where it's combined with other natural compounds to make it work even better. (See the *Foods, vitamins, and minerals chart* on page 351.)

❖ **Eat for your allergies.** In addition to eating fresh fruits and vegetables chock full of vitamin C, here are more allergy-fighting foods to enjoy.

- Dark green and sweet peppers contain vitamin B6, an excellent allergy fighter.
- Asparagus, spinach, nuts, and seeds contain vitamin E, another natural antihistamine.
- Yogurt and other cultured milk products lower the allergens in your digestive tract.
- Green tea makes vitamin C work better and strengthens your immune system.

❖ **Exercise the right way.** Certain sports are better than others for keeping your allergies at bay. Outdoor sports such as hiking, running, horseback riding, and in-line skating are more likely to put you on the road to an allergy attack. Swimming, weight training, indoor aerobics, and bowling are good choices for healthy, allergy-free exercise.

❖ **Avoid the obvious.** If you know your Aunt Sara's smoking really bothers your sinuses, don't visit her when your allergies are acting up. Stay away from spray paint, insect sprays, and magic markers with toxic fumes. Instead, choose latex paint in a can, insect strips or roach motels, and watercolor markers that won't make your allergies worse. Avoid the irritating fumes of dry cleaning by wearing more washable clothes. When clothes come home from the cleaners, hang them outside or in a ventilated garage for a few hours to let the fumes evaporate.

❖ **Stamp out interior allergens.** Vacuum your house twice a week to remove dust and dust mites, pollen, and animal dander. You may want to get some of the new super-filtering vacuum bags that are available. Dust regularly in the out-of the-way spots you might forget, such as under the refriger-ator, behind the sofa, and on the blades of the ceiling fan. Check your kitchen, bath, and base-ment for damp places where mold, another power-ful allergen, can grow. Wipe it out with a solution of bleach and water. Limit your indoor garden to just a few plants. The wet soil of houseplants can grow a bumper crop of mold.

❖ **Garden wisely.** If you're a gardener, make your yard and garden beautiful with plenty of non-allergy-causing plants. Usually, plants with bright flowers don't cause problems for allergy sufferers, so they're a good choice for landscaping. The cul-prits are most often weeds, grass, and trees.

Trees that are likely to cause a pollen prob-lem are ash, birch, cottonwood, elm, oak, olive, pecan, poplar, walnut, and willow. Better choices for people with allergies are dogwood, fig, fir, mag-nolia, palm, pear, pine, plum, and tulip trees. The shrubs to avoid if you have allergies are elderber-ry, juniper, and privet. Allergy-free choices for your outdoor space include boxwood, nandina, pyracantha, verbena, viburnum, and yucca.

Being able to see the world around you is a precious gift. Take good care of your eyes by looking out for illness or injury that could rob you of of your sight. If your eye problems are limited to allergies, try our self-care tips to keep yourself comfortable and better able to see eye-to-eye with the world.

Face pain

Dull, throbbing, or sharp, piercing pain on one or both sides of the face or forehead

"My face hurts!" "Yeah, well, it's killin' ME." While this may be a snappy comeback for a stand-up comedian, it's not so funny if you are among the millions of Americans who suffer from aches and pain in your face, forehead, or jaw. If you can rule out a facial injury, tension headache, and even depression as a cause of the pain, you still have a long list to choose from. Face pain falls under three main categories: nerve disorders, referred pain, and infection.

Nerve disorders

 It's time to see your doctor if you have face pain and:

- Intense, pounding headache on one or both sides of your head
- Scalp tenderness
- Swelling, soreness, and lumps along the temporal artery (blood vessel in the temple)
- Vision loss — from partial to complete blindness
- Low fever
- Loss of appetite
- Aching muscles and fatigue

Because many of these symptoms resemble the flu, sufferers may not go to their doctor right away, but if you are over 50, you must get medical attention immediately. You may have temporal arteritis or polymyalgia rheumatica, similar diseases that inflame the arteries over the temple. You can go blind if you don't get treatment.

- Ache in or near one ear
- Total or partial paralysis of the muscles on one side of the face
- Drooping eyelid and mouth on the affected side
- No expression on affected side of the face
- Loss of sense of taste
- Change in hearing
- Uncontrolled tearing and inability to close the affected eye

These symptoms indicate you may be suffering from Bell's palsy, an upsetting but not life-threatening condition. Bell's palsy strikes when a facial nerve swells, probably from a viral infection, and stops working properly. This condition can be treated, so see your doctor.

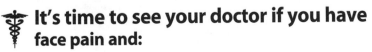

Effects of Bell's Palsy

- Intense, stabbing pain on one side of the face, affecting the cheek, lips, gums, or chin
- Pain lasts a few seconds to several minutes and becomes more frequent over time
- Triggers for the pain can be chewing, washing, brushing teeth, touching, shaving, drinking, talking, or even a breeze

These unusual symptoms could mean you suffer from trigeminal neuralgia, or tic douloureux, which means "painful twitch." This disorder affects the trigeminal nerve that controls the face, teeth, mouth, nose, and jaw. There is no known cause for this nerve damage, but a doctor can treat the pain and decide if you need to see a neurologist.

Referred pain

⚕ It's time to see your doctor if you have face pain and:

- Crushing pain in the middle of the chest
- Pain that spreads to the shoulders, neck, teeth, jaw, back, or arms
- Fatigue

- Lightheadedness, faintness, and shortness of
    breath
- Sweating
- Nausea
- Fever

If you have these signs, you may be having a heart attack. Although the symptoms can range from mild to severe, you should not hesitate in getting immediate medical attention.

- Heavy tightness, aching, burning, or squeezing in
    the chest or between shoulder blades
- Difficulty breathing, or choking feeling
- Pain may spread to jaw or teeth
- Left arm, hand, shoulder, or elbow aches, tingles,
    or feels numb and heavy
- Pale face and sweaty brow

These symptoms could mean you are suffering from angina pectoris. You have an angina attack when your heart does not get enough oxygen, usually because of coronary heart disease. This is not a heart attack. See your doctor immediately, however, and consider the attack a warning sign — you are at risk of a heart attack. (See also *Chest pain* chapter.)

- Headache
- Soreness in jaw muscles
- Clicking or popping noises when opening or clos-
    ing your mouth
- Jaw pain when yawning
- Difficulty opening your mouth completely
- Jaws that lock open or closed

These symptoms could be caused by temporomandibular joint syndrome (TMJ), a spasm of the jaw muscles. Bad habits, such as clenching or grinding your teeth, emotional stress, injury, and even an incorrect alignment of your teeth can cause TMJ. (See also *Jaw pain* chapter.)

- Sudden and intense pain in and around your eyes
- Nausea and vomiting

- Foggy or blurred vision
- Halos around lights
- Eye redness
- Dilated or enlarged pupil

Acute glaucoma is a rare but serious condition. See your doctor immediately.

Infections

☤ It's time to see your doctor if you have face pain and:

- A stuffy nose with a green-yellow discharge
- Tension, fullness, pain, or pressure in your face and head
- Loss of sense of smell
- Fever and chills
- Cough and sore throat

Your sinuses are air-filled pockets and passageways in the bones around your nose that connect your nose, eyes, and ears. When your sinuses become irritated and inflamed by allergies, pollution, smoke, or a viral infection, you can develop sinusitis. (See also *Nose, runny or stuffy* chapter.)

- Ache or throbbing pain in a tooth
- Swollen, red, and sore gum around tooth
- Swollen and tender glands in neck and side of face
- Earache
- Fever
- Bad-tasting discharge in your mouth

Bacteria sometimes reach the nerves and blood vessels inside a tooth, or the area between the teeth and gums, causing an infection. If this infection spreads into the tissue and bone surrounding the tooth, an abscess develops. See your dentist as soon as possible.

- Fever and chills
- Several days of skin sensitivity or tingling along one nerve path anywhere on the face or body
- Burning or shooting pain along the affected nerve

> Blistery, red, itchy rash which turns dry and
> crusty after a few days

These are the symptoms of herpes zoster, more commonly known as shingles.

Immediate help for shingles

Did you have chicken pox as a kid? If so, you remember the pain and itchiness, and were probably relieved to learn you could only get chicken pox once. And technically that is true, but a case of shingles will feel very much like that childhood illness — only worse. That is because shingles is caused by the same virus.

The virus that causes chicken pox can lie in the nerves of your spine for years, decades even. Then, usually after age 50, the virus may become active again if you suffer an illness that lowers your body's immune system. If you have Hodgkin's disease, leukemia, or AIDS, or have received an organ or bone marrow transplant, you're definitely at risk. But sometimes, something as simple as stress or the common cold can trigger the virus.

A case of shingles is much more painful than chicken pox because the herpes zoster virus attacks your nerves. The blistered area will follow the path of the infected nerve, most often along your ribs, back, or side, but sometimes on your shoulders, arms, or face. If the blistery rash affects your eye, it may damage your cornea, and you could lose your sight temporarily or permanently.

After running the course of symptoms, shingles will most often clear up by itself. It is, after all, a virus. But that doesn't mean you have to just lie there and take it. It is severely uncomfortable, so you need to take an active role in your recovery. This will relieve your feelings of helplessness.

❖ **Hands off.** Just like they told you when you had chicken pox — don't scratch. You don't want to break open the blisters. They are full of the shingles virus, and spreading them will only prolong your discomfort. Cut your fingernails and consider wearing gloves or mittens to bed. You may undo all your good intentions by scratching in your sleep.

❖ **Soak the itchies away.** Fill the tub with warm water and sprinkle in any of the following: one to two cups of Aveeno powder, one-half to one cup of baking soda, one to two cups of finely ground (colloidal) oatmeal, or one cup of cornstarch. Soak for 20 minutes.

❖ **Try some anti-rash recipes.** There are many products you can gently apply to the rash to help relieve the itching and dry up the blisters. Calamine lotion and Caladryl are both found in your local pharmacy. Other soothers you may try are aloe vera gel, hydrogen peroxide, or even apple cider vinegar.

❖ **Some like it hot.** Moist compresses, laid gently on the rash, may relieve your pain and itching. Doctors say to use whatever temperature makes you feel better, warm or cool. If you prefer a cold pack, try wrapping a bag of frozen peas in a thin towel. Sometimes, pouring ice water over the towel-wrapped area is easier to tolerate.

❖ **Take a pill.** Don't overlook the simple remedy of aspirin, ibuprofen, or acetaminophen. If needed, your doctor can add a narcotic to your prescription. You might also find relief from a low dose of an antidepressant that would limit pain signals to the brain. Over-the-counter antihistamines will dry up the sores and maybe make you drowsy enough to sleep comfortably.

❖ **Come in from the cold.** Chilling your skin, whether you're outdoors or in, makes it contract and shiver. This can make the itching worse. So stay out of those snappy breezes and air-conditioned drafts.

❖ **Get rid of the gauze.** Doctors recommend leaving the shingles blisters uncovered as much as possible since air promotes drying and healing. Bandages tend to stick to the sores anyway, causing even more discomfort.

❖ **Get out of bed.** While you may feel like moping around feeling sorry for yourself, it is important to stay active, both mentally and physically. And lying in bed may actually irritate your rash. So do that crossword puzzle, or keep up with a hobby. Your mind will stay off the pain, and the time will pass more quickly.

❖ **Care for your kisser.** If you develop blisters in your mouth, you will have to be especially gentle during your daily routine. Use a baby toothbrush, eat soft foods, and gargle with saltwater.

❖ **Pursue that little virtue called patience.** When you are in the middle of an illness like shingles, the symptoms may seem endless. But the condition usually clears up in about three to five weeks. If you don't have the misfortune to develop another condition called postherpetic neuralgia (PHN), you'll soon be your old self again.

The long-range plan for shingles

If you are over 60 and had a severe rash with the herpes zoster virus, you have a strong chance of developing postherpetic neuralgia. With PHN, you continue to feel pain for weeks or even years after your shingles attack because the virus has badly damaged your nerves. Unfortunately, it is difficult to treat.

❖ **Pass the pepper, please.** An over-the-counter cream containing capsaicin (Zostrix) is actually made from hot red peppers. It works by lowering your skin's sensitivity to heat and pain. While capsaicin helped more than half of the PHN sufferers in a recent study, not everyone can tolerate it. Check with your doctor before using it and make sure all the initial shingles blisters are healed.

❖ **Modern medicine or quack cure?** Due to the severity of PHN pain, many sufferers will try anything. There are several treatments, such as electric currents, injections, and neurosurgery, that have not been proven effective. However, antidepressants, acupuncture, self-hypnosis, and biofeedback may give you some relief. Discuss any procedure with your doctor.

❖ **Think positive.** Many doctors insist that optimism brings about better results than any medical treatment.

Research continues in the battle to treat herpes zoster, or shingles. The National Institutes of Health and other clinics and laboratories around the world are working hard to learn more about this common virus. Take heart that the next few years will see an effective treatment to relieve the severe pain and suffering this virus causes.

Face rash or flushing

Sudden redness of the face and/or neck
Eruption of spots or patches on the face, usually
*   temporary*

Years ago, young girls would pinch their cheeks for a rosy glow. But what happens if you are the shy type that blushes easily and often? It's not as simple to hide unwanted redness.

A blush from heat or emotion is just your body's way of responding to a stimulus. The tiny blood vessels in your face and neck expand, and the blood flow becomes more noticeable. It's nothing you can control, and nothing you should really worry about. However, sometimes illness or fever causes your facial redness. This calls for more serious attention.

☤ It's time to see your doctor if you have face flushing and:

Rough patch of skin on cheek, nose or forehead
Extensive sun exposure

139

Painless, scaly patches like this may mean you have a pre-cancerous condition called actinic keratosis. The scalp, face, ears, lips, arms, and hands are especially susceptible to the sun's harmful UV rays since they get so much exposure. Actinic keratosis is a warning sign of skin cancer, so don't ignore it.

- Fever
- Swelling on neck

These are the symptoms of rubella. See a doctor immediately.

- Fever
- Dry cough
- Sore, red eyes
- Runny nose
- Sore throat
- Headache

You could have come down with any number of viral infections, from the measles to Rocky Mountain spotted fever. See your doctor to be sure.

- Small blisters (sometimes)
- Burning feeling on your skin
- Dizziness
- Nausea or vomiting
- Have been in the sun recently

This is more serious than a simple sunburn. You may be extremely sensitive to the sun, a condition called photosensitivity. You and your doctor should try to discover if any medications or skin products are causing this.

- Itching
- Use a prescription drug

Call your doctor immediately. You may be having a reaction to medication.

- Itching

    Light-red bumps with raised edges that enlarge
        and spread quickly

You may be suffering from hives, an allergic reaction
to food, heat, cold, insect bites, animals, medication, or something else. Get to a doctor to determine the cause of the reaction. The hives may
disappear within hours, or may last much longer.

    Itchiness or pain in the affected area
    Flakiness or blistering

This kind of rash may be your body's reaction to
an irritating substance. It is a kind of allergy
called contact dermatitis. The most common causes are detergents, nickel in jewelry, cosmetics,
plants (such as poison ivy), and cleansers.

    Redness on the cheeks, nose, chin, or forehead
        that begins as occasional flare-ups, but gradu-
        ally becomes more permanent
    Swollen, red, bumpy nose
    Burning, irritated eyes
    Oily skin/pimples

These symptoms could mean you suffer from
rosacea (rose-AY-see-uh), a skin disease that is
often misdiagnosed as adult acne. It is important
to distinguish between the two conditions because
causes and treatments are different.

The long-range plan for rosacea

Rosacea normally is not a teenage condition. Sufferers
most often develop symptoms in their 30s or 40s, and
even after turning 50. An estimated 13 million
Americans suffer from rosacea, and that number is
growing as the population ages. While not a life-threatening illness, the physical effects of the disease can be
quite harmful, both emotionally and socially.

Doctors don't know what causes rosacea, but if you
blush easily, you're more likely to develop it. It's possible
that your top layer of skin has thinned or weakened so
much that you can actually see the tiny blood vessels
underneath.

141

Rosacea also may be hereditary. It most often affects fair-skinned adults of Irish, English, Scottish, Scandinavian, or East European ancestry. Women tend to develop rosacea, while men are more likely to suffer from rhinophyma, a swelling of the nose. If you repress your emotions, experience hormonal changes, or have sensitive skin, you're also more likely to get the disease.

Many people mistake the early signs of rosacea for sunburn, and because the symptoms come and go in cycles, they tend to put off treatment. But rosacea will not go away by itself and, if left untreated, will leave your face scarred for life.

Although rosacea cannot be cured, it can be controlled, but you must take an active role in its treatment. Dermatologists do not recommend you do it all yourself, however, since many over-the-counter remedies are designed for acne, not rosacea, and will make the condition worse. Ultimately, a dedicated combination of professional treatment and lifestyle changes is the only way to see improvement.

Your dermatologist can prescribe several methods of treatment. The most common and most successful are oral antibiotics and antibiotic gels or creams for your face. Although this approach takes patience and commitment, 70 to 80 percent of rosacea sufferers see a great improvement. You may opt for more drastic treatments, such as laser surgery to reduce the noticeable blood vessels, or dermabrasion to scrape off the top layer of skin.

The most important thing you can do is to write everything down. Keep a diary pinpointing when your face gets flushed and what activity or substance provoked it. Each time your face flushes, it makes your overall condition more permanent and severe, so it is important to avoid it as much as possible. Most triggers fall into six categories: food and drink, emotional influences, temperature and weather, exercise, drugs, and body products.

❖ **Eat, drink, and be careful.** Avoid spicy foods and hot drinks. They make the blood rush to your head, causing you to blush. Some rosacea sufferers have problems with certain fruits, especially citrus; vegetables like beans, spinach, and avocados; and dairy products. And while rosacea is not related to alcoholism, alcohol can make a case of rosacea worse.

❖ **Check your stress.** Anxiety apparently is the number one cause of rosacea flare-ups, so avoid worry and tension whenever possible. Relax, breathe deeply, and find the joy in life. This does not mean, however, that you should suppress your feelings of anger or fear. That can be just as bad.

❖ **Your weatherman is your friend.** Most rosacea sufferers say summertime is the worst time. Heat, sun, and humidity are major triggers of flushing. So to make it through the hot months, protect yourself when you go outdoors by wearing a hat and a facial sunscreen of Sun Protection Factor 15 (SPF 15). Schedule your outdoor activities in the early morning or evening to avoid the worst of the day's heat. And use any strategy to keep cool. Keep a fan running in the kitchen when the oven is on; place a cool, damp cloth around your neck; or relax with a tall glass of iced tea or lemonade. Unfortunately, winter can bring its share of problems as well. Cold weather and wind can whip a healthy glow into your cheeks, but it's not a welcome sight if you have rosacea. A hat and scarf will help protect your face from the frigid temperatures, and don't forget to wear a moisturizer.

❖ **Exercise with caution.** You must maintain a regular exercise routine for general health and a sense of well-being, but as a rosacea sufferer, use common sense. Begin with low-level activity and set your own pace to avoid becoming overheated. Around the house or yard, watch out for those little jobs that require lifting or moving heavy objects. A sudden burst of exertion can cause more blood to rush through your body. And avoid those after-exercise saunas or hot baths. Even though your aching muscles may benefit from the heat and steam, your skin won't.

❖ **What's in that pill?** Certain drugs are vasodilators, which means they will cause your blood vessels to

Living with lupus

Your body's immune system is like a police department, ever vigilant against disease-causing microorganisms. When the police attack innocent citizens, such as your lungs, kidneys, or skin, you have what is called an autoimmune disorder. Lupus, or systemic lupus erythematosus, is such a condition. Latin for "wolf," lupus was first named for the face rash that resembles a wolf's bite. Today, it is more common to hear it referred to as a butterfly rash.

Many experts believe lupus is hereditary but activated by outside factors such as stress, infections, exposure to sunlight, injury, surgery, exhaustion, or certain drugs and chemicals. The disease is not as rare as it was once thought, afflicting more than half a million Americans, mostly women.

Diagnosing lupus is difficult, since it resembles many other disorders and can attack any part of your body. Along with a rash, symptoms include weight and hair loss, fatigue, poor circulation in fingers and toes, abdominal and chest pain, and arthritis. The symptoms come in different combinations, and may disappear for weeks, months, or even years.

Once your doctor has positively identified lupus, don't despair. The disease may not be curable, but it can be treated and, with some minor adjustments, you should be able to lead a normal life. Help yourself by learning stress management and relaxation techniques, getting plenty of exercise, and also enough rest. To protect yourself from the sun, wear hats, sunglasses, sunscreens, and long-sleeved clothing.

relax and get larger. They are used in the treatment of a wide variety of heart and vascular (blood vessel) conditions. The most commonly prescribed drugs are amyl nitrite, cyclandelate, dipyridamole, ethaverine hydrochloride, isoxsuprine hydrochloride, nimodipine, papaverine hydrochloride, and tolazoline hydrochloride. Ask your doctor or pharmacist if any of your medications are vasodilators.

❖ **Be gentle to your skin.** Try to avoid these ingredients in skin care products: fragrance, alcohol, menthol, eucalyptus oil, witch hazel, peppermint, clove oil, acetone substances, and salicylic acid. Your rule should be water soluble, gentle, and natural. Anything that stings, burns, or causes redness will aggravate the problem.

When cleansing your face, be gentle. Don't rub too hard or massage it. This stimulates blood circulation and will cause even more redness. Rinse with lots of cool water and blot dry. If you have a prescription medication from your doctor, pat it on gently and allow to dry. Many rosacea sufferers have found that a green-tinted makeup covers the redness remarkably well. Check with your doctor before using any other moisturizer, sunscreen, or makeup to be sure they will not react with your medication. Remember that part of the treatment of rosacea is looking and feeling your best.

Soap, moisturizers, and makeup are not the only products to examine either. Perfumes, aftershave lotion, shampoo, hair spray, and even household products like laundry aids, can contain irritants.

Suffering from rosacea does not have to change your life. You should only have to make slight changes in your habits or routine to control your symptoms. Moderation is the key word, and isn't that the secret to a longer, healthier life?

Faintness and weakness

Sudden feeling of overwhelming fatigue
Feeling too weak to function normally
Feeling that you are about to faint

Feeling strong and energetic is the gift of a healthy body, no matter how young or old you are. You need a certain amount of energy just to get up in the morning and begin your day, and you need energy and momentum to carry you through your normal activities. But if your day is interrupted by periods of feeling faint or weak, you can lose your momentum and end up feeling like a deflated balloon.

A number of different conditions can be at the root of your energy crisis. Constant anxiety can eat away at your energy and leave you feeling tired and weak. When taken to extremes, worry and anxiety can result in a panic attack that leaves you faint, weak, and shaken. A temporary drop in blood pressure is normal after a big meal, but it can make you feel faint and weak if you jump up quickly from the dinner table. And faintness and weakness are common side effects of both prescription and over-the-counter drugs.

Mild faintness and weakness often occur without indicating any real problem. But they may be pointing to some condition for which you need to see your doctor, especially if they go along with the following symptoms.

 ## It's time to see your doctor if you have faintness and weakness and:

- Exposure to hot weather without drinking enough fluid
- Cramps in your muscles
- Very rapid or very slow heartbeat

These are the signals of heatstroke or heat exhaustion. Too much heat has built up in your body, and it is not able to cool down. This is a medical emergency, so get help immediately. (See also *Muscle cramps or weakness* chapter.)

- Recurring headache
- Nausea and vomiting
- Breathing problems

These symptoms signal carbon monoxide poisoning, usually from some kind of heating system, engine, or industrial fumes. You must find the source of the carbon monoxide and fix it. Carbon monoxide poisoning can cause death. (See also *Headache* chapter.)

- **Irregular heartbeat that feels like a fluttering in your chest**
- **Breathing difficulty**
- **Tiredness**

You may have atrial fibrillation, in which your heart beats irregularly and too fast. Your heart may feel as if it's flopping around in your chest. This type of irregular heartbeat may resolve itself, but it is usually dangerous if left untreated, so you need to see your doctor.

- **Sudden fatigue**
- **Extremely slow heartbeat (60 or fewer beats per minute)**

These are the symptoms of bradycardia, or slow heartbeat. With this condition, your heart may slow down too much and just stop beating. Bradycardia is normal in a well-conditioned athlete, but not in most other people. It may mean you have an underlying disease, or your heart medicine (such as a beta-blocker) is slowing your heart rate too much.

- **Shortness of breath or difficulty breathing, especially when lying down**
- **A cough that is worse when you lie down**
- **Wheezing**
- **Rapid or irregular heartbeat**
- **Low blood pressure**
- **Swollen legs, ankles, and feet**

These symptoms could mean you have developed a heart complication, called congestive heart failure, as a result of another disease or illness. High blood pressure, heart attacks, emphysema, or various infections can cause the heart to stop pumping as strongly as it should. Blood backs up into other organs, especially the lungs and liver, and these symptoms appear.

147

- Appetite loss
- Yellow eyes and skin
- Nausea, diarrhea, vomiting
- Low-grade fever (less than 101° F)
- Pain or discomfort in upper abdomen

Liver problems are a likely source of your symptoms. You may have cirrhosis of the liver, viral
hepatitis, or liver cancer. See your doctor immediately.

- Tiredness
- Appetite loss
- Darkening of skin, freckles, scars, and breast
  nipples
- Low blood pressure, causing dizziness or faintness
  when you stand up
- Vomiting, diarrhea

Your symptoms could add up to Addison's disease,
a condition your doctor can control with hormone
treatments. If you experience pains, feel faint, have
low blood pressure, or a high or low temperature,
get help immediately. You may be having an adrenal
crisis, which can be fatal if not treated promptly.

- Fatigue
- Pale skin

These symptoms could indicate you have some type
of anemia, due to a lack of iron, folic acid, or vitamin B12 in your diet. (See the *Food, vitamin, and
mineral chart* on page 351.)

- Unexplained weight loss
- Anxiety/hyperactivity
- Rapid, irregular heartbeat
- Always feel warm or hot
- Bulging eyes

You may be suffering from hyperthyroidism, also called
thyrotoxicosis, toxic goiter, or Graves' disease. This is a
relatively common disorder caused by an overactive
thyroid. It can usually be controlled by medication.
(See also *Weight changes, unexplained* chapter.)

148

- Extreme hunger
- Headache
- Sweating, nervousness
- Dizziness, confusion
- Rapid heartbeat
- Drowsiness

These symptoms could be caused by hypoglycemia, or low blood sugar. This means your body doesn't have enough energy to keep up with all its activities. The condition may result from diabetes, an over-active pancreas, a reaction to certain drugs, or even another condition. See your doctor for an accurate diagnosis.

Immediate help for hypoglycemia

Your body needs fuel to run, just like a car. But instead of gas, your body's systems run on glucose, a simple form of sugar. The hormones insulin and glucagon control the amount of glucose in your blood. When you don't have enough glucose to fuel your body's activities, you end up with hypoglycemia, or low blood sugar.

If you have diabetes, you already know the signs of hypoglycemia. Weakness, hunger, sweating, and confusion are sure signals that your insulin level is out of balance and your blood sugar is too low. You also know you should do something quickly to raise your blood sugar, like drinking orange juice or eating hard candy, or you might be heading for big trouble.

What if you don't have diabetes but still get the symptoms of hypoglycemia? You may have nondiabetic hypoglycemia, which could be caused by several underlying conditions, or sometimes by an unknown factor. Or you may just be extra-sensitive to changes in your blood sugar level. Some doctors think this kind of hypoglycemia is a forerunner to diabetes.

The immediate treatment is still the same. If you have that faint and weak feeling, you need to get something into your body that will raise your blood sugar to a normal level. If you don't have any fruit juice or candy at hand, try one to two cups of milk, two to three tablespoons of sugar stirred into a glass of water, a piece of fruit, some crackers, or a piece of cake. Once your blood sugar is back to normal, eat a healthy meal with some protein included to ward off another hypoglycemia attack.

The long-range plan for hypoglycemia

That awful, sinking feeling of hypoglycemia can hit you at any time. If you are constantly surprised by it, try keeping a record of the circumstances surrounding the episode — what you were doing and what and when you ate before it happened. In both diabetic and nondiabetic people, hypoglycemia can be brought on by too much exercise, going too long without food, or drinking too much alcohol. If you take beta blocker medications, exercise is more likely to bring on hypoglycemia. People who are alcoholics or binge drinkers often have hypoglycemia. You can even get hypoglycemia from a Jamaican fruit called ackee if you eat it before it's ripe.

Some medical problems also cause low blood sugar. Liver disease, kidney failure, hormone or enzyme deficiencies, some cancers, and tumors of the pancreas can all make you shaky and dizzy. Pancreatic tumors are usually benign and can be successfully treated with surgery.

If you're older, you may show much different symptoms than someone younger than you. Depression, confusion, dizziness, incontinence, falling, weight loss, and paranoia are some of the frightening symptoms you might experience.

If you are diabetic, hypoglycemia can be life-threatening. If you're not diabetic, recurring hypoglycemia may not be life-threatening, but it can make your life complicated and unpredictable. It can also put your body under constant physical stress. Here are some things you can do to prevent unpleasant attacks of hypoglycemia.

❖ **Don't leave home without it.** A snack, that is. Carry hard candy or glucose tablets (available at your local drugstore) to help in a sugar crisis, but also carry a snack to eat at the proper time so you won't have to deal with hypoglycemia.

Crackers with peanut butter or cheese, a piece of fruit, or half a sandwich should do the trick.

❖ **Organize your eating.** For people with hypoglycemia, the best way to eat is in small doses. Eating five or six small meals a day instead of three big ones will keep your blood sugar on a more even keel.

❖ **Try more protein.** This is a controversial area, but some people find that a diet high in protein and moderate to low in carbohydrates successfully treats hypoglycemia. Others advocate a diet high in unrefined carbohydrates. Either way, you should eat lots of fresh fruits and vegetables and stay far away from refined carbohydrates such as sugar and white flour. Save the candy and sweets for emergencies only.

❖ **Be careful of caffeine.** Caffeine heightens the effects of hypoglycemia. If you've just had a big meal of carbohydrates and not much protein, a cup of coffee can bring on the symptoms of hypoglycemia. It's best to reserve caffeine for the times when you're also eating protein, or avoid caffeine after a high-carbohydrate meal.

❖ **Exercise safely.** If you tend to get hypoglycemia, you need to take special care when you exercise. Take a snack and emergency food (glucose tablets, candy, or fruit juice) just in case you need them. Try to exercise with a friend if possible, and be sure she knows the signs of hypoglycemia and can help you if necessary.

Watch out for the conditions in your life that can leave you feeling faint and weak. The biggest factor is one you have control over — your diet. What and when you eat can influence the level of sugar in your blood, and the level of energy in your life.

Fatigue

A tired feeling
Inability to perform usual physical activities

You've been working in your yard all day, mowing, raking, and weeding. When you're finished, all you want to do is collapse on your sofa from exhaustion. That type of fatigue is normal and no reason for concern.

But if you're tired all the time, your body is probably trying to tell you something. You may simply have a vitamin deficiency and need to eat a more balanced diet or take supplements. You may have a viral or bacterial infection, or suffer from energy-draining stress or depression. Numerous medical conditions, including cancer, can cause fatigue. If your fatigue is interfering with your normal daily activities, or if you have other symptoms, don't just take a nap, take a drive to your doctor's office, and get some answers.

It's time to see your doctor if you have fatigue and:

- Excessive thirst
- Increased appetite
- Frequent urination
- Unexplained weight loss

These symptoms may mean you have diabetes. (See also *Weight changes, unexplained* chapter.)

- Appetite loss
- Yellow eyes and skin
- Nausea, diarrhea, vomiting
- Low-grade fever (less than 101° F)
- Pain or discomfort in upper abdomen

Liver problems are a likely source of your symptoms. You may have cirrhosis of the liver,

High blood pressure — hidden cause of fatigue

If you can't find a reason for your tiredness, consider hypertension, or high blood pressure. It has few outer symptoms, but headache and fatigue could be warning signs. High blood pressure is a serious health problem because it increases your risk for stroke and other diseases. Have your pressure checked immediately if you suspect it might be high.

If you have high blood pressure, here are some steps you can take to bring it down without the use of drugs.

❖ **Reduce your salt intake.** This step alone should lower blood pressure for more than half the people who have it.

❖ **Lose weight if you are overweight.** Cutting the amount of fat in your diet, plus a healthy exercise program, are the best ways to slim down.

❖ **Reduce your alcohol intake.** Be sure it's less than three drinks a day. Limiting it to just one is even better.

❖ **Increase your fiber.** Doctors say your diet should contain 25 to 30 grams of fiber a day. Raw fruits and vegetables and whole grain cereals and breads are excellent sources of fiber.

❖ **Ease some magnesium into your diet.** This mineral may help reduce blood pressure and improve heart health. Spinach, baked potatoes, black-eyed peas, and sunflower seeds are high in magnesium.

❖ **Increase carbohydrates.** Eat only the healthy complex ones found in potatoes, rice, and other grains. Cut out the sugary treats.

❖ **Get some garlic.** This old remedy can actually lower high blood pressure.

viral hepatitis, or liver cancer. See your doctor immediately.

- Appetite loss
- Darkening of skin, freckles, scars, and breast nipples
- Low blood pressure, causing dizziness or faintness when you stand up
- Vomiting, diarrhea

Your symptoms could add up to Addison's disease, a condition your doctor can control with hormone treatments. If you experience pains, feel faint, have low blood pressure, or a high or low temperature, get help immediately. You may be having an adrenal crisis, which can be fatal if not treated promptly.

- Shortness of breath or difficulty breathing, especially when lying down
- Irregular or rapid heartbeat
- Cough
- Swollen stomach, legs, and ankles

Together, these symptoms may indicate congestive heart failure, which is usually a complication of other illnesses such as heart or lung disease.

- Breathing difficulty
- Pale skin

These symptoms could mean you have some type of anemia, due to a lack of iron, folic acid, or vitamin B12 in your diet. (See the *Food, vitamin, and mineral chart* on page 351.)

- Unexplained weight loss
- Anxiety/hyperactivity
- Rapid, irregular heartbeat
- Always feel warm or hot
- Bulging eyes

You may be suffering from hyperthyroidism, also called thyrotoxicosis, toxic goiter, or

Graves' disease. This is a relatively common disorder caused by an overactive thyroid. It can
usually be controlled by medication. (See also
Weight changes, unexplained chapter.)

- Chest pain
- Weight gain or loss
- Sleepiness or insomnia
- Depression or poor memory
- Decreased sweating, appetite, and tolerance for
    cold

These symptoms might indicate hypothyroidism,
an underactive thyroid. Although hypothyroidism
is generally easy to treat with thyroid replacement
drugs, it can cause life-threatening complications
in rare cases, so it is important to see your doctor.
(See also *Weight changes, unexplained* chapter.)

- Sore throat
- Fever
- Achy, run-down feeling

If you have these symptoms, you may have
mononucleosis, a viral infection spread mostly by
saliva (which earned it the nickname "kissing disease"). It is especially common among college students.

- Weakness
- Forgetfulness or confusion
- Joint or muscle pain
- Mood swings and/or depression

If your fatigue is persistent, and you have the
above symptoms, you may have chronic fatigue
syndrome.

Immediate help for chronic fatigue syndrome

You've always been a cheerful, energetic person,
always on the go, always willing to help out a friend.
Now, however, you just can't seem to summon up much
energy. You're too tired to work, too tired to play, and

155

Feeling the pain of fibromyalgia

"Where does it hurt?" We often ask children that question, but if your answer would be, "Here, and here, and here, and here ...," you may have fibromyalgia. The fatigue this disease causes is accompanied by achiness, stiffness, sleep problems, bowel problems, swollen hands and feet, and headaches. It is a poorly understood disorder, confusing to both patients and doctors. Since no test can reliably identify fibromyalgia, The American College of Rheumatology has established guidelines for diagnosis, including identifying 18 tender spots located in pairs throughout the body. If you have pain in at least 11 of these, along with widespread pain for three months or more, you could have fibromyalgia.

Research has not yet found a cause or an easy cure for this disease. Regular aerobic exercise helps relieve some of the pain and stiffness, and your doctor may prescribe painkillers or medication to help you sleep. Guaifenesin, an ingredient in many cough syrups, is thought by some to reverse fibromyalgia. Unfortunately, it makes the pain worse before it gets better. If you decide to try it, be sure to avoid products containing salicylates, such as aspirin and Alka Seltzer, because they will interfere with guaifenesin's healing ability.

For help in dealing with fibromyalgia, contact the Arthritis Foundation, 1314 Spring St., N.W., Atlanta, GA 30309 (404) 872-7100, or call your local chapter. They can send you a pamphlet on fibromyalgia and give doctor referrals.

you're depressed and confused. Concerned friends urged you to go to the doctor, so you did. He poked and prodded and tested for several different conditions. The tests all came back normal, but you're still exhausted. Maybe you have Chronic Fatigue Immune Dysfunction Syndrome (CFIDS) or what is commonly called chronic fatigue syndrome.

CFIDS is difficult for doctors to diagnose because the symptoms mimic so many other conditions. However, once those conditions have been ruled out, CFIDS may be the answer. If your fatigue has persisted or recurred for six months or more, and you can do less than half of what you could before, you may have CFIDS. Other symptoms include mild fever, confusion, concentration problems, sore throat, muscle aches, and sleep problems.

CFIDS often begins after you have had an infection like a cold, bronchitis, or mononucleosis. No one knows for sure what causes it, but most doctors now believe a virus, such as herpes, sets it off. Most people who have CFIDS carry some form of the herpes virus. Researchers think this virus may lay dormant in your body until extreme stress or an illness weakens your immune system and lets CFIDS take over.

Because no one is sure what causes chronic fatigue, it is difficult to treat. Doctors usually treat specific symptoms. For instance, many doctors prescribe antidepressants to treat the depression that often accompanies CFIDS. This works well for many people. Your doctor also may prescribe medicine to help you sleep better, so you wake feeling a little more refreshed and energetic.

Although CFIDS has no cure, some lucky people find their symptoms disappear on their own after a few months. For others, the battle with fatigue rages on and off for years.

The long-range plan for chronic fatigue syndrome

You may not be able to cure your chronic fatigue, but you can help control it. The first step is to recognize you have the disorder. The media labelled chonic fatigue the "yuppie flu" a few years ago because most reported cases involved well-educated, middle class women. Many people, including some doctors, believed it was not a legitimate illness. Although CFIDS is becoming a more accepted (and more common) diagnosis, it is sometimes still taken very lightly. However, CFIDS can change your life, making you unable to work or function as well as before. If you realize you have CFIDS, you can take steps to make sure this syndrome doesn't take over your life as well as your energy.

❖ **Regular, mild exercise.** Many people who have CFIDS find their energy level sometimes rises.

When this happens, they tend to work or play very hard to make up for lost time and to take advantage of their fleeting energy. However, they often pay for their overexertion with sore muscles. Exercise can help the symptoms of CFIDS, but you need to exercise a little restraint as well. Don't overdo it when you're feeling well, and try to keep up with mild exercise even when you're tired. Ask your doctor to help you choose exercises that are appropriate for your abilities and energy level.

❖ **Write it down.** Keep track of your daily activities and note the times you seem to have the most energy. If you have peaks and valleys of fatigue at regular times, you may be able to plan your day around the times when you are most likely to be feeling well.

❖ **Get some support.** Chronic fatigue can be draining, not only physically, but emotionally as well. Check into local support groups for CFIDS, try some counseling, or just lean on your family and friends. Because CFIDS is so difficult to diagnose, some people need to be reassured that their illness is not "just in their heads."

❖ **Diet right.** While there is no magical dietary formula for CFIDS, a few dietary guidelines may help you become more energized. Eat plenty of fruits, vegetables, and complex carbohydrates. Many people with CFIDS are prone to allergies, so identify foods you may be sensitive to, and avoid them. You should also avoid or limit your intake of alcohol, caffeine, sugar, nicotine, and aspartame (Nutrasweet).

❖ **Increase your vigor with vitamins.** When you are ill for a long time, your body often uses up extra amounts of vitamins, creating a deficiency. This could be the case in CFIDS. A multi-vitamin supplement may provide you with the extra vitamins you need, especially the B vitamins, which help your body turn protein and other nutrients into energy.

❖ **Lysine may lighten your load.** Lysine is an amino acid supplement that may help clear up cold sores from the herpes virus. It may prevent your body from absorbing another amino acid called arginine, which helps the herpes virus reproduce. Since most people with CFIDS carry some form of the herpes virus, lysine may control the virus and make you feel better. One to two grams of lysine daily is the recommended dosage. If you decide to take lysine supplements, be sure to avoid foods that contain arginine, such as nuts, chocolate, raisins, whole wheat, brown rice, and cereal. They'll work against your efforts to control the herpes virus.

Despite researchers' efforts, chronic fatigue is still a mystery illness. But as the syndrome affects more and more people, the chances are greater that researchers will find a cause and a cure. In the meantime, take heart in knowing you are not alone, and if others have found a way to live with chronic fatigue, so can you.

Foot pain

Aches, pain, or tenderness in the toes, arch, instep, or heel

Your feet are the unfortunate victims of fashion, foul play, and foolishness. How many times have you squeezed into stilettos, sideswiped the sofa, or stomped on a splinter? Yet your feet always come through for you; perhaps a bit battered, but still functional. It isn't until something goes seriously wrong with your feet that you realize just how much you need them in good working condition.

 It's time to see your doctor if you have foot pain and:

- A recent injury to your foot
- Pain or tenderness
- Bleeding or bruising
- Numbness, tingling, or paralysis
- You can't put weight on your foot
- No pulse in your foot

It is possible you have fractured a bone in your ankle or upper foot. As you age, your bones become thinner and more brittle. Even a slight injury can break one of the small bones in your foot. Don't delay seeing a doctor, especially if you experience foot numbness, tingling, or loss of pulse. Setting a bone becomes much more difficult after six hours.

- Exposed skin becomes numb, hard, and white
- When warmed, the area tingles or burns and becomes red and swollen
- Blisters and gangrene in severe cases

Frostbite occurs when parts of your body are exposed to subfreezing temperatures. The cold slows down your blood flow, and body tissue can actually freeze. (See also *Hands and feet, cold and tingling* chapter.)

- Leg cramps
- Chest pain
- Headache
- Dizziness

With these symptoms, you may have atherosclerosis, a condition in which fat builds up on your artery walls and restricts blood flow. More commonly known as "hardening of the arteries," atherosclerosis is a major cause of fatal heart disease and stroke in the U.S. (See also *Impotence* chapter.)

- Redness, tenderness, and swelling, especially around the big toe
- Severe pain that usually occurs at night

Gout is a form of acute arthritis marked by inflammation of the joints. It usually begins in the knee or foot and is caused by too much uric acid in the

Diabetic (peripheral) neuropathy

Diabetic neuropathy is a nerve disorder caused by diabetes. If it affects the legs, feet, arms, and hands, it is known as peripheral neuropathy. The symptoms include tingling and numbness in your hands, feet and legs; loss of balance and coordination; shooting pains that are worse at night; pale, dry, and sensitive skin; and weight loss.

The nerve damage from this condition can affect your reflexes, muscle response, and pain reaction. The last problem is a major concern, because if you don't feel pain, you can injure yourself without knowing it. Your feet are at special risk because the nerves to your feet are the longest in your body, so they are the ones it affects most often.

Here are some general health tips you can use to help fight and control this condition:

- Stop smoking. It increases circulatory problems and the risk of neuropathy and heart disease.

- Alcohol also can make neuropathy worse.

- Work with your doctor on an exercise routine. Staying fit can lessen the pain of neuropathy as well as improve your body's circulation, muscle tone, and use of insulin. Avoid exercises such as running or aerobics.

- Control your body's blood sugar by eating healthy foods, low in fat and sugar.

blood, which forms crystals in the joints. Attacks usually last about a week.

- **Morning stiffness**
- **Limited movement and dexterity**

This could mean osteoarthritis, a condition where the cartilage in your joints gradually breaks down. Usually, you will feel an aching pain when you move or put weight on your joints. (See also **Knee pain** chapter.)

- Swelling, redness, and stiffness in your foot or ankle
- Pain in your ankles, arches, and toes
- Low fever
- General ill-feeling

These symptoms may signal the onset of rheumatoid arthritis, a disease that inflames the joints.

- Small, hard growth on the bottom of your foot
- Pain when you walk

You probably are suffering from a plantar wart. The virus that causes these kinds of warts is passed from one person to another, so see your doctor for treatment and advice on preventing a recurrence.

- Burning pain
- Small blisters
- Foot odor
- Itching and inflammation
- Scaly patches on your feet, especially between your toes

These symptoms are most likely caused by athlete's foot, a contagious foot fungus that infects the skin of your feet. You can buy over-the-counter treatments, but if you have a severe case, your doctor will prescribe more powerful antifungal medications.

- Stiffness in your toe joints
- A swollen area at the base of the big toe where the skin has thickened
- Your big toe curves inward, sometimes overlapping the second and third toes

You may have a bunion. If you have a family history of bunions, suffer from arthritis, or have spent many years wearing ill-fitting shoes, you are more likely to develop one yourself. Your doctor can tell you how to keep the bunion from becoming worse, and in extreme cases may prescribe surgery to remove the bunion and improve the placement of the bones in your foot.

Pain under the heel bone

If you run or jog, have a job or recreational activity that requires a lot of standing, or are overweight, you are at risk of developing a heel spur, a hard growth in the muscle below the heel bone.

A weight problem

If you are more than 20 percent over the recommended weight for your age, sex, and height, you are clinically obese. Besides being at risk for a multitude of general health problems, you can also suffer strain-related difficulties with your feet, ankles, and knees.

Sharp pain on the bottom of your foot, near your heel
Pain is worse in the morning

Plantar fasciitis occurs when the rubber band-like tissue on the bottom of your foot becomes inflamed or torn. This usually results from strain caused by certain types of exercise, or simply changes in its elasticity due to aging.

Immediate help for plantar fasciitis

Heel pain affects nearly two million people every year. That's a lot of sore feet. Experts say, however, that you should try self-treatment for at least two weeks before going to a doctor. In most cases, simple exercises and over-the-counter remedies will do the trick.

❖ **Go shoe shopping.** Check the fit of your shoes. Do they pinch, rub, or strain your calf muscles? Do they support your arches properly? Flexible soles with good cushioning are vital if you spend a lot of time on your feet or walking on hard surfaces. Remember that saying, "as comfortable as an old pair of shoes"? Well, in many cases that is a dangerous notion. Just because your running shoes started out comfortable two years ago doesn't mean they're still doing the job you bought them for. Just like anything else, support can wear out.

❖ **Insert some comfort.** You can buy custom-made shoe inserts, called orthotics, and pay anywhere from $200 to $400. In some cases, the cost would be warranted. But for under $50, you can get over-the-counter silicone heel cushions, heel cups, felt heel pads, or arch supports, and receive the same pain relief. It can't hurt to try the easier, less expensive method first and see if you're satisfied.

❖ **Flex and point.** By giving some special attention to your feet, you can gradually strengthen the foot muscles and relieve your pain at the same time. Do these exercises twice a day.

● Place a golf ball on the floor and gently roll your foot over it.

● With both knees slightly bent, place one foot flat on the floor behind you. Bend your front knee more, straightening your back leg and keeping your back heel on the floor. Move your heel gently up and down to feel the stretch in your back foot. Repeat with the other leg.

● Stand facing a wall. Place your heel on the floor and your toes up on the wall. Gently stretch your heel and the bottom of your foot as you push against the wall.

● Sit with one leg straight out in front of you. With any long, flexible piece of rubber, hook the toe part of your outstretched shoe and pull gently back toward you as you push your foot against the tubing.

Protecting your feet from neuropathy

If you have peripheral neuropathy, take these special precautions to keep your feet injury-free:

❖ Check your feet every day. Look for cuts, sores, redness, swelling, bumps or bruises. Call your doctor at the first sign of infection.

❖ Wash your feet carefully in warm water, but do not soak them, as this softens up any protective calluses you may have. Test bath water with your wrist or elbow. Dry your feet thoroughly, especially between your toes. Use lotion to keep the skin from cracking.

❖ Wear soft, white cotton socks. This will make it easier to see blood or fluid from cuts or blisters. Don't wear socks with holes or seams and avoid stockings.

❖ Buy shoes that fit you correctly, without pinching or rubbing. Break new shoes in slowly, wearing them for only an hour at a time. When trying shoes on, allow for any swelling your feet may have near the end of the day.

❖ Check your shoes daily for debris inside or tears that could irritate your feet.

❖ Never go barefoot.

❖ Trim your toenails straight across, never rounding the corners. Make sure no nail is rubbing against another toe.

❖ When you sit, prop your feet up, and periodically rotate your ankles and wiggle your toes. Do not sit with your legs crossed since this restricts circulation. Get up and walk around every once in a while.

❖ Have your doctor check your feet at each visit.

● Scrunch up a towel with your toes as if you're going to pick it up. (See picture on previous page.)

❖ **Soak your troubles away.** Five to 10 minutes in warm water will loosen your muscles and soothe your aches. Follow up with a gentle massage, and you'll be in foot heaven.

The long-range plan for plantar fasciitis

With some thoughtful changes to your lifestyle, you can reduce the likelihood of suffering from muscular problems like plantar fasciitis.

❖ **Check your weight.** Added pounds place added stress on your feet and ankles. If you can maintain an ideal body weight, you will be less likely to have foot problems.

❖ **Golf anyone?** Sports or recreational activities that involve foot stress, high foot impact, or stop-start movements can cause painful conditions like plantar fasciitis. Consider something gentler.

When you think about how much stress and abuse your feet take, it is amazing how well the tiny bones and ligaments hold up. Throw in a lifetime of standing, walking, and fashionable shoes, and you have a recipe for trouble. But by thinking about your feet a little more carefully, you can prevent problems before they begin.

Forgetfulness

The inability to remember

You go to the grocery store for milk and come back with bags full of groceries ... but no milk. You meet someone on the street who greets you warmly by name, and you hate to admit it, but you don't have a clue what his name is. This type of forgetfulness is annoying and sometimes embarrassing, but it doesn't mean there is anything wrong with you. It is probably just a by-product of your busy life.

Sometimes, however, long periods of forgetfulness can signal a physical or emotional problem. If you forget the name of your spouse or child, or forget important facts — like where you live — you may need to see your doctor. He can help you determine the cause of your memory problems.

Stress, anxiety, and just not getting enough sleep can cause your memory to become a little fuzzy. Prescription drugs can sometimes cause forgetfulness as a side effect. See your doctor, and if he determines that you're healthy but just forgetful, you may have to resort to the old trick of tying a string to your finger. Of course, then you'll have to remember why you tied the string there.

⚕ It's time to see your doctor if you have forgetfulness and:

- Seizures
- Speech problems
- Nausea or vomiting
- Confusion/dizziness
- Severe headache
- Loss of vision or visual disturbances

These symptoms could mean you have a brain tumor. See your doctor immediately for a diagnosis.

- Anxiety/confusion
- Mood swings
- Loss of appetite
- Difficulty sleeping
- Thoughts of death or suicide
- Feelings of sadness or hopelessness
- Lack of enjoyment in activities or life in general

Depression is a common condition, especially as you age. Physical problems, such as an illness, medication, or hormonal changes, can bring it on. So can social or psychological factors. Don't feel you have to fight it alone. Get help as soon as possible. (See also *Depression* chapter.)

- Persistent fatigue
- Weakness
- Joint or muscle pain
- Mood swings and/or depression

If you have the above symptoms, you may have chronic fatigue syndrome. (See also *Fatigue* chapter.)

- Headache
- Dizziness
- Slurred speech
- Blurred vision or double vision
- Weakness in your arms or legs

You may be experiencing a transient ischemic attack (TIA), which is a temporary brain disturbance that usually clears up within 24 hours. It is also possible you have had a mild stroke. See your doctor immediately. (See also *Slurred speech* chapter.)

- Shivering
- Sluggishness
- Difficulty controlling hand movements

If you have been exposed to extremely cold temperatures, you may be suffering from hypothermia, which means your body temperature is dangerously low.

- Depression
- Anxiety
- Sleep problems
- Personality changes
- Trouble finding the right words to express yourself

These symptoms may mean that you are in the early stages of Alzheimer's disease.

Immediate help for Alzheimer's disease

You've searched high and low for your car keys, and you finally find them — in the microwave oven. Now you're standing, car keys firmly in your grasp, but you can't remember where you had planned to go. This type of forgetfulness is common in people with Alzheimer's disease, and it makes life difficult for the person with the disorder and for their family. Sometimes it can even be dangerous, if a person forgets to turn off the stove or stop at a red light.

Alzheimer's disease was discovered almost a century ago by a German doctor, but it has probably affected people for much longer. People with Alzheimer's were considered senile or just crazy in years past, but now we know it's a specific disease that clouds your mind — not just normal aging.

Think of a water hose with a kink in it, blocking the water from coming out at the end. The same thing happens when your brain cell connections block up, but in your case it's information flow that stops. For example, you may be trying to think of a word. You know what it is, but if the pathway to your mouth is blocked, the word will never reach your lips.

What blocks your brain cell connections? Tangled strands of fibers and worn out areas called plaques seem to be the problem. Researchers have found them in the brains of Alzheimer's sufferers and are studying them further to discover how and why they form. Only then can they figure out how to prevent them.

Although no one knows what causes Alzheimer's, researchers do know that certain people are more likely to get the disease. Your single biggest risk factor is age. Alzheimer's affects five to seven percent of people over age 65, and about 20 percent of the people over age 80. You are also more likely to get Alzheimer's if you have a relative with the disease.

Although research has not yet found a cure for Alzheimer's, doctors can prescribe medicine to help relieve symptoms. The FDA recently approved a new drug for the treatment of the disease. In clinical trials, 80 percent of the people with Alzheimer's who took Donepezil HCl (Aricept) improved mentally or at least did not decline while they were taking the drug. Medical advances like these give hope that someday soon Alzheimer's will be a disease of the past.

The long-range plan for Alzheimer's disease

Alzheimer's usually takes over a person's life very slowly. You may misplace things or forget appointments, grope for words, or find that you suddenly can't balance your checkbook. In the later stages of the disease, you may be unable to care for yourself at all. But you're more likely to die from other causes before you reach the more serious stages of this disease. Doctors won't know if you actually have Alzheimer's unless they perform an autopsy and find the tell-tale plaques and tangles.

Although Alzheimer's has no cure as yet, promising research is sure to unlock the mystery of this disease soon. In the meantime, take advantage of the knowledge we do have to keep this disease from striking you.

❖ **Find brain protection in your medicine cabinet.** Researchers study the people most likely to get Alzheimer's for clues to curing this disease. They also notice who is least likely to get it, such as people with rheumatoid arthritis. Since arthritis sufferers usually take daily doses of nonsteroidal anti-inflammatory drugs (NSAIDs), like aspirin and ibuprofen, researchers guess those drugs might protect them from Alzheimer's. They think brain inflammation may cause the plaques found in Alzheimer sufferers, and anti-inflammatories protect the brain from developing these plaques.

❖ **Go with gingko.** The leaves of the gingko tree may help shade you from Alzheimer's. Extracts made from this tree have been used for centuries for a variety of ailments, including brain problems. Research finds that gingko increases blood flow, and more blood flow to your brain may help make it work better. At least one scientific study found that symptoms improved significantly in people with Alzheimer's who took 240 mg of gingko daily.

❖ **Puzzle over it.** If you love to work crossword puzzles or fit the pieces of a jigsaw into place, you may be less likely to get Alzheimer's. Whenever you learn something new or exercise your brain, your brain cells make new connections. Studies show that the more connections you have, the less likely you are to get this disease. Of course, you don't have to stick to puzzles; any type of mental exercise will create and strengthen those connections.

❖ **Education counts.** Education may help you succeed financially by making it easier to get a well-paying job. Education may also help you avoid Alzheimer's, probably because of the extra connections it creates between brain cells. If you didn't finish eighth grade, you're twice as likely to get Alzheimer's as those who have more education. If you also work at an unchallenging job, you're three times more likely to develop the disease.

❖ **Connect emotionally.** Brain cell connections play an important role in Alzheimer's. Emotional connections may do the same. A strong relationship with your spouse may not prevent you from developing Alzheimer's, but it may make it less severe, and maybe even help you live longer. It also may keep you out of a nursing home. Studies find you're less likely to be institutionalized if your spouse cares for you, rather than a nurse or other relative. Without positive emotional support, many Alzheimer's sufferers may simply give up and let the disease take over.

❖ **Add some antioxidants.** Getting plenty of antioxidants in your diet, like vitamins A and C, may help protect you from Alzheimer's. Antioxidants fight free radicals, which are unstable molecules in your body that damage your cells. Research finds that people with Alzheimer's have taken in fewer antioxidants in their lifetimes than people without the disease.

❖ **Replace your estrogen.** Many women decide to use estrogen replacement therapy (ERT) to keep the symptoms of menopause at bay. However, researchers have discovered that ERT may do more for you than just cool down your hot flashes. It may help prevent Alzheimer's from stealing your memories. One study found that only 2.7 percent of the women who took estrogen developed

Alzheimer's compared with 8.4 percent of those who didn't.

Everyone forgets things once in a while, and being a bit absent-minded does not mean you have a serious condition. Although aging involves some normal slowing down, studies have shown your brain can remain as sharp and creative as a 25-year-old's if you keep it active and challenged. A little mental workout each day is all it takes to keep you alert and fit well into your golden years.

Gum bleeding

Bleeding in the soft tissue surrounding your teeth

If the thought of a trip to the dentist makes you break into a cold sweat, you're not alone. Just remember that it's less painful, not to mention less costly, if you take care of your teeth before something goes wrong. Your dentist can monitor your general oral health, which is sometimes the first place other problems show up. If your gums begin to bleed, check your mouth for an injury or cold sore. If you wear dentures, be sure they fit properly and are not rubbing. Once you eliminate all the easy answers, you need to consider other possibilities.

 It's time to see your doctor if you have gum bleeding and:

- Fever
- Bleeding from your nose
- Bruising
- Bone tenderness
- Headache, stomach pain
- Enlarged lymph nodes and spleen
- Repeated infections in your chest, throat, skin, or mouth

Leukemia is a type of cancer that affects the production of white blood cells. Your doctor can study a sample of your bone marrow to determine if you have the disease. Acute leukemia comes about more suddenly than chronic leukemia but has a fairly high survival rate.

- Red or purple spots on the skin
- Nosebleeds
- Bruising
- Blood in the urine
- Heavy vaginal bleeding
- Headaches or dizziness (sometimes)

Thrombocytopenia is a long word that means you don't have enough platelets in your blood. Platelets are the tiny disks that join to stop bleeding. If you don't have enough platelets, your blood is unable to clot, so you bleed more heavily and often. There are many possible causes and treatments of thrombocytopenia, and recovery is high. You need to see a doctor for an accurate diagnosis.

- Blood spots under the skin
- Unexplained bleeding from your nose, intestinal or urinary tract
- Slow clotting
- Bruising

If you lack vitamin K, you may show signs of these symptoms. Certain bacteria in your intestines make this vitamin, which the liver uses to produce blood-clotting substances. Without enough vitamin K, you will bleed more than usual. (See also *Bruising, unexplained* chapter.)

- Bad breath
- Teeth and gums hurt when you eat food that is cold, hot, or sweet
- Intense pain when chewing on one side of your mouth
- An unpleasant taste in your mouth

173

These symptoms point to periodontitis, an infection in the tissues that hold your teeth in place. See your dentist as soon as possible to avoid complications from this gum disease, such as tooth loss or an infection in your bloodstream.

- Fatigue
- Bleeding from your nose, gums, rectum, or other areas
- Unexplained bruising
- Sores in the mouth, on the tongue or rectum

You could be suffering from aplastic anemia, a condition where your bone marrow does not produce enough blood cells. This is usually treatable, so see your doctor immediately.

- Bad breath
- Inflamed gums that are red, soft, and shiny

If you have these symptoms and your gums bleed when you brush your teeth, you probably have gingivitis, an infection in your gums. This is a treatable problem, but one you shouldn't ignore. Left unchecked, gingivitis can lead to periodontitis, a more serious stage of gum disease.

Immediate help for gingivitis

Even though gum disease is uncommon in people younger than 30, it affects about 90 percent of Americans over age 65. Gingivitis stems from poor oral hygiene and is preventable. You simply need to take good care of your teeth and gums.

❖ **Brush.** Twice a day is standard fare for most people, but adding a toothbrush session after any sweet or sticky snack makes good dental sense. Use a soft toothbrush and small circles, paying particular attention to the gum line, where most plaque grows. Hold the bristles at a 45-degree angle to your teeth. Choose a fluoride toothpaste, but pass on the baking soda. Many experts say baking soda is too abrasive and can scour the protective enamel right off the tooth surface. You should spend at least two minutes brushing to really clean your teeth — a small investment in a healthy smile.

❖ **Floss.** Use waxed or unwaxed dental floss at least once a day to clean between your teeth. Gently scrub the floss up and down around each tooth.

❖ **Swish.** Read mouthwash labels and choose one that fights plaque. Prescription mouthwashes containing chlorhexidine seem to be effective in preventing gingivitis. In studies, this germ-killing mouth rinse reduced some bacteria by 50 percent. Ask your dentist if you should use this product.

❖ **Chew.** Saliva is your mouth's first method of plaque assault, since it rinses food particles from your teeth. So unwrap that stick of sugarless gum and chew, chew, chew. You'll increase your saliva as you do.

The long-range plan for gingivitis

In most cases, gingivitis is reversible. A good program of regular dental care is all it takes to get your teeth and gums in tip-top shape. Once you achieve a healthy mouth, concentrate on keeping it that way.

❖ **Make a date with your dentist.** Some people get yearly checkups, but having a professional cleaning every six months is even better. See your doctor more often if you suffer from any type of gum disease.

❖ **Eat well.** A varied diet of nutritious foods will prevent vitamin deficiencies and improve your health all around. Avoid sticky, sugary foods since these coat your teeth and promote decay.

❖ **Kick the habit.** If you smoke, you are five times more likely to develop gum disease than if you don't.

❖ **Expose the plaque.** You can buy "disclosing tablets" at your grocery or drug store. Chewing one will stain any plaque on your teeth red. This shows how well you've brushed.

175

Vitamin C deficiency

Vitamin C is an important ingredient in your body's mix of nutrients. Also known as ascorbic acid, it plays an essential role in maintaining healthy bones, teeth, gums, ligaments and blood vessels; helps fight infections and heal wounds; and helps your blood absorb iron. If your body is low on vitamin C, you'll show the following symptoms:

❖ Unexplained bruising

❖ Confusion

❖ Nosebleeds

❖ Loss of teeth

❖ Rough skin

❖ Weakness

❖ Swollen, occasionally bleeding gums

❖ Hallucinations or odd behavior

❖ General aches and pains

Poor nutrition is the major cause of vitamin C deficiency. If you've been ill, are on a fad diet, or have simply changed your eating habits, you may not be eating a balanced diet. Other causes include hyperthyroidism, a serious burn or injury, or recent major surgery. Oral contraceptives or exposure to cigarette smoke can reduce your vitamin C levels as well.

Fixing the problem is as easy as eating a healthy mix of fruits and vegetables. Foods with the highest vitamin C content include papaya, green or red peppers, oranges, pink grapefruits, kiwi, and cantaloupe. You should also munch on foods from the cabbage and greens families, as well as plenty of tomatoes, potatoes, strawberries, and pineapple. (See the **Food, vitamin, and mineral chart** on page 351.)

Be careful not to over-compensate and take massive doses of vitamin C supplements, as this may cause other problems. Your doctor can evaluate the cause of your deficiency and recommend the proper treatment.

Hand and wrist pain

Sharp or aching pain in hand or wrist
Tingling, numbness, or weakness

"Honey, would you open this jar for me?" This request may make your spouse feel strong and needed, but if you have pain in your hands or wrists, it probably makes you feel frustrated. Your hands stay so busy during the day, you don't even think about how vital they are ... until pain interferes with simple tasks like opening jars or doors. Pain, numbness, or tingling in your hands or wrists can affect all areas of your life and sometimes may be a symptom of a larger problem.

It's time to see your doctor if you have hand and wrist pain or numbness and:

- Tingling or numbness in your hands and feet
- Seizures
- Muscle cramps or weakness

These symptoms, along with an irregular heartbeat, may signal that you have too little calcium in your blood. This is a medical emergency, and you should get help immediately.

- Morning joint stiffness
- Limited movement and dexterity

This could mean osteoarthritis, a condition where the cartilage in your joints gradually breaks down. Usually, you will feel an aching pain when you move or put weight on your joints. (See also ***Knee pain*** chapter.)

177

- Tight, thick, shiny skin (especially on fingers and face)
- Raynaud's phenomenon (hands and feet become red, white, and blue when exposed to cold)
- Difficulty swallowing
- Heartburn

These are symptoms of a rare but potentially fatal disease called scleroderma. It is a condition where your immune system attacks your own tissues. In mild cases, it affects only your skin, but severe cases may involve your heart, lungs, kidneys, gastrointestinal tract, and joints.

- Knots in your palm, usually at the base of your fingers

These type of knots could signify Dupuytren's disease, which occurs mostly in older people. In this condition, nodules develop in your palm, often causing your fingers to bend involuntarily inward.

- Swelling
- Warmth in affected area
- Muscle pain or tenderness that increases with motion

If you have these symptoms you may have tendinitis, an inflammation of your tendons. The problem often is caused by an injury or by repeating the same motion over and over. (See also *Arm, elbow, or shoulder pain* chapter.)

- Pain is located mainly in your thumb, index, and middle fingers
- Pain is worse at night
- Weakness in your thumbs
- Numbness or loss of feeling in fingers

These symptoms could result from a condition known as carpal tunnel syndrome.

Immediate help for carpal tunnel syndrome

What do typists, meat cutters, jack hammer operators, computer operators, and sign language interpreters

178

have in common? They sound like a pretty diverse group, but they're all alike in at least one way. They are at greater risk for developing carpal tunnel syndrome.

This condition mainly affects people whose work requires repeated motions with the hands and wrists. You don't have to be in one of the above professions to be affected, though. Many activities can cause it, even enjoyable ones like needlework or playing the piano or guitar. Occasionally, it occurs for no apparent reason.

You have several nerves which allow you to move and feel your hands and fingers. One of them — the median nerve — runs through an area in your wrist called the carpal tunnel. Tendons, which connect your muscles and bones, also pass through this tunnel. If you overuse these tendons, they may swell and press on the median nerve. Since that nerve controls feeling and movement in your hand, the result will be pain, numbness, or tingling throughout your hand and wrist.

Anti-inflammatories like ibuprofen may give you short-term relief. If your pain persists, your doctor may recommend shots of corticosteroids.

The long-range plan for carpal tunnel syndrome

Though your kids may accuse you of living in the Stone Age, there's really no doubt you are living in the Information Age. Computers are now an important part of modern life. Simply click on the Internet, and you can find all types of information, chat with people thousands of miles away, play games, and even shop. But does all this convenience come with a price? Can "surfing the net" be hazardous to your health?

Unfortunately, it might. The more we use computers, the more we develop stress injuries like carpal tunnel syndrome. Carpal tunnel is not a new disorder — it was once called the illness of knitters. Today, however, it is more likely to be chalked up to the hazards of computer use. But if you are a typist, computer operator, or dedicated net surfer, don't despair. You can take steps to protect your hands from this painful, numbing condition.

- ❖ **Sit correctly.** "Sit up straight! Don't slouch," your mother used to tell you. Mom was right once again. Sitting incorrectly can lead to carpal tunnel and other problems, especially if you're in front of a keyboard all day long. Make sure your chair and keyboard are at a comfortable height for you, and don't slump over. Sit up straight or lean back slightly.

- ❖ **Straighten your wrists.** If you work at a keyboard, don't rest your wrists on your desk. When you do this, you bend your wrists upward, which increases your risk of carpal tunnel. If you have a problem holding your wrists straight, buy specially made wrist rests for your keyboard.

- ❖ **Brace yourself.** Wearing a wrist brace may help keep your wrists straight so they don't put constant pressure on your median nerve. If this interferes with your work, try wearing the brace only at night, which is when much of the pain occurs anyway.

- ❖ **Take a break.** If you are doing anything that requires repeated hand movements, take a break every hour or so. Do something different for a few minutes to relieve the stress on your hands.

- ❖ **Shake it out.** Some people find temporary relief by shaking or rubbing their hands. If your pain occurs at night, try hanging your hands over the side of the bed while you sleep.

- ❖ **Beware of B6.** Some health professionals believe a vitamin B6 deficiency may cause carpal tunnel syndrome. However, a recent study found no connection, and large doses of B6 can cause permanent nerve damage. Make sure you get enough vitamins, but be careful if someone recommends megadoses of B6 for this condition.

- ❖ **Lighten up.** If you are overweight, you are at greater risk for carpal tunnel. Losing weight will help your hands, your heart, and your overall health.

If these suggestions don't help, discuss your condition with your doctor. He may recommend surgery to relieve pressure on the median nerve. But don't put it off, hoping the problem will go away. Without treatment, your nerve damage, along with your painful symptoms, may become permanent.

Hands and feet, cold and tingling

*Toes or fingers that are painfully affected by the cold
A tingling sensation in hands and feet*

We have all experienced "pins and needles" when we have sat too long in one position or fallen asleep with an arm at an odd angle. And who hasn't worn socks to bed on a cold wintry night? But when these symptoms combine and occur more than just occasionally, the result can be troubling. Many people never associate these signs with any larger issue, but they can mean something more serious.

 It's time to see your doctor if you have cold and tingling hands and feet and:

- Weakness
- Dizziness
- Confusion
- Blurred vision
- Difficulty speaking

These are all warning signs of a stroke. Do not waste time. Call your doctor immediately. (See also *Slurred speech* chapter.)

- Weakness and fatigue

181

> Frequent urination

These symptoms indicate a possible disorder of the endocrine system, which includes your pituitary glands, thyroid, pancreas, adrenal glands, ovaries or testicles.

> Weakened muscles
> Shooting pains at night
> Ulcers on your toes or fingers
> Pale, dry and sensitive skin
> Weight loss

If these symptoms gradually appear over several months and spread throughout your body, you might have peripheral neuropathy, a disease of the nerves. This can result from a reaction to drugs or chemicals, or it could be a complication of another problem such as diabetes. It is important to identify the cause and correct it if possible. (See also *Foot pain* chapter.)

> Weakness on one side of your body
> Recently lifted something heavy or engaged in vigorous exercise

It is possible you have ruptured a disk in your back. (See also *Back pain* chapter.)

> Stiff neck
> Headaches
> Dizziness
> Double vision
> Slower reflexes
> Pain in your neck, shoulders or upper arms
> Cracking sounds when you move your neck or shoulders

Arthritis of the neck can affect many areas of the body. Your doctor can help you decide on the best way to relieve your symptoms. (See also *Joint pain* chapter.)

> Muscle spasms or cramps
> Seizures

- Irregular heartbeat
- High blood pressure

Something as simple as too little calcium in your body can trigger a whole host of nasty symptoms. Calcium supplements can easily remedy this problem.

- Sharp pain in your hand or arm, especially at night
- Cramped, stiff hands in the morning
- No recent injury
- Cannot make a fist
- Drop objects often

This could mean you suffer from carpal tunnel syndrome, a common complaint from people who work repetitively with their hands. (See also *Hand and wrist pain* chapter.)

- Take a prescription drug

Many drugs can cause adverse reactions or side effects.

- Your fingers turn white then blue when cold
- When warmed, they turn red and may throb and swell
- Pain and numbness as your fingers change colors
- Attacks that last minutes or hours
- Infections around your fingernails and toenails
- Ulcers on your fingers and toes

These symptoms could signal Raynaud's disease. This is a disorder of the circulatory system that restricts the amount of blood flowing to the fingers and toes. Sometimes the ears and nose are affected as well.

Immediate help for Raynaud's disease/phenomenon

If you have Raynaud's disease and go out in the cold, the blood vessels in your hands and feet will contract more than they should. Less blood reaches your fingers and toes, and they feel cold, tingly, and numb. If you don't treat the condition, and your hands and feet are deprived of enough oxygen, ulcers and gangrene can set in.

Raynaud's disease can occur for no apparent reason, or it can result from other conditions. If this is the case, it is called Raynaud's phenomenon. Raynaud's disease is actually quite common. It occurs more often in women than men and usually begins to develop before age 40.

❖ **Swing those arms.** A few minutes of large, vigorous circles will increase the blood flow to your hands and fingers.

❖ **Protect your hands and feet.** Wear double layers on your hands and feet when you're outside in cold weather. Woolen socks, mittens, and insulated boots will hold in a layer of warm air. Indoors, be aware of the simple ways your hands might touch something cold. Drink beverages from an insulated glass, or wrap a napkin around a cold can or bottle. Use tongs to get ice from the freezer, or keep an old glove handy and slip it on when you need to dig out those frozen steaks. Avoid vibrating machines like chain saws which place a lot of stress on the hands and arms. And never abuse your hands by using them instead of an appropriate tool.

❖ **Adapt your activities.** Your day undoubtedly is filled with activities that can chill your hands. When cooking, washing dishes, or cleaning, use tepid water instead of cold, or pull on a pair of rubber gloves. Have you ever backed out of the driveway on a wintry morning? The steering wheel can feel like a ring of ice. Why not heat up the car a few minutes early or insulate the cold vinyl with sheepskin covers? Gardening can be a wonderfully relaxing activity but not if you're digging in chilly spring dirt. Wait for a sunny time of day, and always wear gardening gloves.

❖ **Exercise carefully.** If you enjoy a brisk walk, a leisurely bicycle ride, or even a round of golf, by all means continue these activities. But when the temperature drops, make sure you protect your whole body with warm, comfortable clothing. Body heat lost through the head, neck, and wrists makes you especially vulnerable to the cold. Also, be careful to stay warm after you stop exercising. That important cool-down period should not make your shiver. Keep a sweatshirt or warm-up suit handy to reduce post-workout chill.

Frostbite

As we age, it becomes even more important for us to stay aware of changes in our bodies. Small differences can mean big adjustments. For instance, our skin becomes thinner as we grow older. That leaves us more susceptible to cold. Our internal machinery slows down and becomes less efficient, so our bodies don't respond to temperature change as quickly. All this means that frostbite can be a real concern during harsh winter months.

Frostbite occurs when parts of our bodies are exposed to subfreezing temperatures. The cold slows down blood flow, and body tissue can actually freeze. Fingers, toes, the nose and ears are most often affected.

What are the symptoms of frostbite? The exposed skin becomes numb, hard, and white. When warmed, the area tingles or burns and becomes red and swollen. Blisters and gangrene can occur in severe cases.

How can you protect yourself from frostbite? Be prepared for changes in temperature. Keep a hat, gloves, scarf, and extra socks handy during a planned outing. Don't drink or smoke before spending time outside in cold weather. Keep moving. Don't sit too long enjoying the winter scenery. It's safer to slow your walk a bit than to stop altogether.

What should you do if you suspect frostbite? Go inside and remove clothing from the affected area. Do NOT massage. Soak the area in warm (not hot) water. Drink something warm with lots of sugar. Don't smoke. If your feet are affected, don't walk. See your doctor.

❖ **Dress for the weather.** Spring and fall are wonderful times to be outdoors, but the weather can be changeable and unpredictable. Too often, we underdress during these transition months and are caught unprepared.

The long-range plan for Raynaud's disease

Unfortunately, Raynaud's disease has no cure. That does not mean you have to let the condition control your life. With a few lifestyle adjustments, you can minimize your discomfort and painful episodes.

❖ **Stop smoking.** Nicotine narrows your blood vessels, restricting circulation. Poor circulation makes it even more difficult for your hands and feet to stay warm. Try to avoid cigarette smoke altogether.

❖ **Relax.** Stress can trigger episodes of Raynaud's disease. Work on removing as many causes of anxiety from your life as possible.

❖ **Avoid drugs that will affect circulation.** Many cold medicines and diet pills contain the drug *phenylpropanolamine* which can affect circulation. Read your labels.

❖ **Try circulatory conditioning.** Don't worry, this is not as hard as it sounds. You are simply trying to "teach" the arteries in your hands to stay open, even when they are cold. When the weather starts to turn cool, sit outside for about 10 minutes with your hands in a bowl of warm water. Do this several times a day, every other day for about a month. This should help you make it through the winter.

❖ **Learn biofeedback therapy.** This will take a little more of your time, but the results can be longer lasting. With professional training, you can learn to control the temperature in your feet and hands, and eventually check attacks of the disease. Not everyone sees improvement, but there are no drug-related side effects.

❖ **Move to a warm climate.** This may seem like a drastic measure, but if your condition is severe

186

enough or simply interfering too strongly with your activities, you may want to consider relocating somewhere with lots of heat and sunshine.

Headache

A sharp, throbbing, or aching pain in your head

If you're searching for relief from headache pain, you're not alone. More than 40 million Americans have chronic headaches and often the pain is severe or disabling. Headache sufferers account for over 8 million visits a year to doctors' offices.

Headaches can be caused by too much sleep, not eating regular meals, stress, poor posture, sinusitis, ear infection, head injury, toothache, and food allergies. Rare causes of headache include high blood pressure; brain tumor; aneurysm, which is a swelling in part of a blood vessel; and inflammation of the arteries of the brain and scalp.

Although nine out of 10 headaches are not life-threatening, some headaches require medical attention.

 It's time to see your doctor if you have a headache and:

- Drowsiness
- Confusion
- Paralysis on one side of your body

If these symptoms follow a head injury, see your doctor immediately. You may have a hemorrhage, or bleeding, in your brain.

- Nausea or vomiting
- Loss of vision or visual disturbances
- Speech problems
- Seizures

These symptoms could mean that you have a brain tumor.

- Breathing difficulty
- Nausea or vomiting
- Weakness
- Cough
- Disturbed vision
- Bleeding in the retinas of your eyes

If you travel to a high altitude, watch out for these symptoms. They may mean you have altitude sickness, which can be very serious. If you are above 10,000 feet and begin to experience a severe headache, confusion or hallucinations, and unsteadiness on your feet, your brain could be starting to swell. This is a medical emergency, so get help immediately.

- Dizziness
- Confusion
- Blurred vision
- Vomiting

If you have recently lost consciousness following a head injury and are experiencing the above symptoms in addition to your headache, you may have a concussion.

- Fever
- Neck stiffness
- Nausea and vomiting
- Sensitivity to light

If you have these symptoms, you may have meningitis, which is an infection of the spinal fluid and the tissues around the brain and spinal cord.

- Blurred vision
- Enlarged pupil
- Teary eye

If your headache pain is dull and located around your eye, you may have glaucoma.

- Stuffy nose
- Fever
- Facial pressure

If you have these symptoms, you may have sinusitis, which is an inflammation of the sinus areas around your eyes and nose.

- **Throbbing pain, usually on one side of the head**
- **Nausea or vomiting**
- **Sensitivity to light**
- **Visual disturbances**

These symptoms may mean that you have a migraine.

Immediate help for migraines

According to Greek mythology, Zeus, the king of the gods, was once stricken with such an intense headache that he bashed his head against a rock. His head split open and Athena, the goddess of wisdom, sprang out. Talk about a splitting headache! The creator of this myth must have been familiar with migraines. The pain and nausea of a migraine headache is sometimes enough to tempt you to bash your aching head against a rock, but that would only make your headache worse. Fortunately, there are real solutions to your pain.

A migraine is a vascular headache, which means it involves changes in blood flow to the brain. For some reason, certain people have blood vessels that react strongly to various triggers. These blood vessels tend to go into spasms in response to triggers such as stress, and they set off a chain reaction of increasing constriction. When these blood vessels constrict and get smaller, the brain receives less oxygen-rich blood.

For some people with migraines, this loss of oxygen to the brain results in an "aura," or a set of warning signals that usually occur before the headache pain begins. Auras usually last about 15 to 30 minutes and involve visual changes. You may lose part of your vision temporarily, or you may see flashes, dots, or zigzags of light. Your body then tries to make up for this loss of oxygen by dilating or widening certain arteries in your brain.

189

5 easy ways to ease a tension headache

❖ **Relax.** Tension headaches usually involve increased tension in the muscles of your neck and scalp. Concentrating on relaxing those muscles may relieve your headache.

❖ **Check your head.** Morning headaches may be caused by depression. Your doctor can determine if your depression is the result of a chemical imbalance. Talking with a counselor, minister, family member, or friend could also help.

❖ **Breathe properly.** Tension headaches can be caused by using your neck and shoulder muscles to lift your rib cage to breathe. Try breathing from your diaphragm, the muscle that separates your chest cavity from your abdominal cavity.

❖ **Posture counts.** Stand up straight. Poor posture can put a strain on your neck muscles and contribute to your annoying headaches. See if your posture passes the test. Stand with your back against a wall. Can you touch your head, heels, buttocks, and the middle of your back to the wall without straining? Can you then slide your hand between the small of your back and the wall? If you can't, or if it's difficult or painful, you need to improve your posture.

❖ **Try some tennis balls.** Take two tennis balls and stuff them into the toe of a nonelastic sock. Lie on your back on the carpet and place the sock under your neck with the balls just under the ridge of your skull. After awhile, your tensed-up neck and scalp muscles should relax, and your headache should just slip away.

This widening causes the release of pain-producing substances called prostaglandins and chemicals that increase your sensitivity to pain. All this adds up to an intense throbbing in your head.

You can take an over-the-counter pain reliever, such as aspirin, for your migraines, but for the best results, you have to take it as soon as your headache begins. If your migraines are severe and interfere with your life, your doctor can prescribe medicine that may help.

If you already have a migraine, try the suggestions below to help ease your pain.

❖ **Remain in the dark.** Many migraine sufferers become very sensitive to light during a headache episode. Draw the shades and turn out the lights for relief.

❖ **Put your headache on ice.** Putting ice packs on your aching head may help reduce the swelling of blood vessels and give you a little relief.

❖ **Put on the pressure.** During a migraine, you may try pressing firmly on the bulging artery that is located in front of your ear on the same side of your head as the pain.

❖ **Drink some java.** Coffee is an old remedy for hangovers. While it may or may not sober people up, it can help prevent the hangover headache. A small amount of caffeine may do the same for people with migraines. Caffeine is a vasoconstrictor, which means that it causes blood vessels to narrow. When the blood vessels in your head are painfully swollen, a little caffeine may be just your cup of tea.

The long-range plan for migraines

If you spend a lot of time in a darkened room with a cold towel over your face, you need a long-term plan for dealing with your migraines. Medicine may help, but if you can avoid getting those sickening headaches in the first place, you'll have more time to enjoy life. Try these suggestions to prevent migraines.

❖ **Identify your triggers.** Migraines may be triggered by emotional factors, such as stress, or environmental factors, like flickering lights or weather changes. Quite often, migraines are triggered by the foods you eat. Scientists believe that certain foods, like yogurt, nuts, and lima beans, contain substances that can cause blood vessels to constrict. Some people have allergies to certain foods that may touch off a migraine. Keep a diary for a few weeks and write down when your headaches strike and what you were doing and eating before the attack. This will help you identify your triggers and avoid them in the future.

❖ **Exercise.** Regular exercise can help reduce the frequency and severity of migraine attacks.

❖ **Try biofeedback.** Biofeedback involves relaxing while mentally directing blood flow away from your head to other parts of your body, like your hands and feet. A biofeedback therapist can teach you how to do this.

❖ **Go fishing.** If you find fishing a relaxing pastime, it may help your migraines by reducing your stress, but eating fish may also help relieve your headache woes. One study found that fish oil capsules containing omega-3 fatty acids reduced the frequency and severity of headaches for 60 percent of the migraine sufferers who participated in the study. You can buy fish oil capsules, or just eat foods containing omega-3 like tuna, cod, salmon, and other seafood.

❖ **Eat at regular intervals.** Low blood sugar may contribute to migraines by causing the blood vessels in your head to dilate. Eating smaller, more frequent meals may help avoid a drop in blood sugar that could set off a migraine.

❖ **Avoid oversleeping.** Sleeping late can also cause a drop in blood sugar that may trigger a migraine, so get up at your regular time, even on weekends.

❖ **Get some herbal assistance.** The herb feverfew has been used to treat headaches for almost 2,000 years. Feverfew contains a chemical called parthenolide that blocks the effects of pain-producing prostaglandins. You can find feverfew at most health food stores, or if you like to garden, you can grow your own. If you buy a commercial feverfew preparation, look for one that contains at least 0.2 percent of the active ingredient parthenolide. If you choose the home-grown route, chew and swallow one or two fresh leaves daily.

Carbon monoxide poisoning: a silent killer

That persistent headache may save your life. Carbon monoxide is a colorless and odorless gas that can kill. You can't see it or smell it, but you can feel its effects. The symptoms of carbon monoxide poisoning include headache, fatigue, chest pain, dizziness, nausea, and confusion. The most common sources of carbon monoxide poisoning are car exhaust and gas appliances in your home.

If you have gas appliances and you are plagued by persistent headaches, call your local utility company and ask them to check your appliances for leaks.

Hundreds of people die each year from carbon monoxide poisoning. Five members of one family in Colorado died after a van was left running in their garage overnight. If you suspect you are suffering from carbon monoxide poisoning, get some fresh air, and call for medical help immediately.

Miners used to take a canary into mine shafts to warn them of silent, deadly gas. That unexplained headache may be all the warning you need to save your life.

Heartbeat irregularity

Fast, pounding heartbeat
Slow, weak heartbeat
Skipping or fluttering heartbeat

Your heart is the powerhouse of your body, an incredible pumping engine that pushes gallons of blood through your veins and arteries every day. A complex system of electrical currents drives your heart to beat in its proper rhythm. When the rhythm slows down, speeds up, or is interrupted, it's called arrhythmia. As you age, you're more likely to develop arrhythmia.

Irregular heartbeats happen every day. Just taking a breath causes your heart to slow down and then speed up again. When you exercise, feel stressed, or get emotionally excited, your heart speeds up. When you relax deeply or sleep, it slows down. You may feel your heart skip a beat occasionally or feel it flutter. It may beat fast and strong for a few moments, a condition known as palpitation. All these heartbeat irregularities happen within a healthy, normal heart and are generally harmless. But others may not be.

If your heartbeat is too slow, too fast, too strong, or too weak, you may have an underlying disease you need to discover and treat.

It's time to see your doctor if you have an irregular heartbeat and:

- Chest pain, heaviness, or tightness
- Pain that radiates from the chest to arms, back, jaw, neck, or stomach
- Sweating
- Clammy skin
- Coughing, shortness of breath
- Nausea, vomiting

These symptoms suggest you may be having a heart attack. Call for help or go to an emergency room or hospital immediately. (See also *Chest pain* chapter.)

- Excessive thirst and urination
- Nausea, vomiting
- Low energy levels
- Constipation

Your symptoms signal that you have too much calcium in your blood. This is an emergency. Get
medical care immediately.

- Tingling or numbness in your hands and feet
- Leg or other muscle cramps or spasms
- Seizures

In this case, you may have too little calcium in
your blood. This also is a medical emergency.

- Very fast or very slow heartbeat
- Weakness and fatigue
- Feeling disturbed and confused
- Paralysis of arms or legs

If this describes your condition, you may have an
imbalance of potassium in your body. This is an
emergency situation; get to a doctor or hospital
immediately.

- It feels like a fluttering in your chest
- Faintness and weakness
- Breathing difficulty
- Tiredness

You may have atrial fibrillation, in which your
heart beats irregularly and too fast. Your heart
may feel as if it's flopping around in your chest.
This type of irregular heartbeat may resolve itself,
but it is usually dangerous if left untreated, so you
need to see your doctor.

- Very slow heartbeat (60 or fewer beats per minute)
- Sudden weakness or fatigue
- Dizziness or fainting

These are the symptoms of bradycardia, or slow
heartbeat. With this condition, your heart may
slow down too much and just stop beating.
Bradycardia is normal in a well-conditioned athlete, but not in most other people. It may mean
you have an underlying disease, or your heart
medicine (such as a beta-blocker) is slowing your
heart rate too much.

- Confusion
- Leg or muscle cramps
- Weakness
- Swelling

These symptoms suggest you may have too little or too much sodium in your blood. Since a sodium imbalance may signal an underlying disorder, see your doctor as soon as possible. (See also *Muscle cramps or weakness* chapter.)

- Decreased sweating, appetite, and tolerance for cold
- Chest pain
- Weight gain
- Sleepiness or trouble sleeping
- Depression/memory problems

These symptoms might mean you have hypothyroidism, an underactive thyroid. Although hypothyroidism is generally easy to treat with thyroid replacement drugs, it can cause life-threatening complications in rare cases, so it is important to see your doctor. (See also *Weight changes, unexplained* chapter.)

- Weakness and fatigue
- Unexplained weight loss
- Hyperactivity
- Generally feel warm or hot
- Bulging eyes

You may be suffering from hyperthyroidism, also called thyrotoxicosis, toxic goiter, or Graves' disease. This is a relatively common disorder caused by an overactive thyroid. (See also *Weight changes, unexplained* chapter.)

- Breathing difficulty
- Fatigue
- Fever
- Chest pain

When these symptoms accompany shortness of breath, they point to myocarditis or pericarditis, an inflammation of your heart or tissues around your heart. This condition can result from illness, surgery, radiation therapy, or a bad reaction to a drug.

- Shortness of breath or difficulty breathing, especially when lying down
- Weakness, fatigue, or faintness
- Cough
- Swollen stomach, legs, and ankles

Together, these symptoms may indicate congestive heart failure, which is usually a complication of other illnesses such as heart or lung disease.

- Tension headaches
- Sweating
- Shortness of breath
- Loss of appetite
- Poor sleep
- Stomach pain
- Have recently undergone a major life upset or change

These symptoms, along with rapid heartbeat, chest pains, and a feeling that something bad is about to happen, often signal stress, general anxiety, or even a panic disorder. These are physical symptoms of an underlying emotional or psychological problem. You need to see your doctor for help in coping with your anxiety. (See also *Anxiety* chapter.)

- Chest pain
- Shortness of breath
- Rapid or pounding heartbeat of 150 to 300 beats per minute
- Feeling that you're going to die

These are the symptoms of rapid heartbeat, or tachycardia.

Immediate help for rapid heartbeat

You're not running a marathon, but just sitting around talking to a friend or snuggling under a warm quilt for an afternoon nap. All of a sudden, your heartbeat takes off at breakneck speed. You are experiencing tachycardia, or rapid heartbeat. It may last for only a few seconds, or it may last for minutes or even hours. If your tachycardia continues for an extended time, it could lead to congestive heart failure or heart attack.

Tachycardia may be a symptom of heart disease, but not always. Sometimes there may not be any underlying cause. You probably don't need to be concerned if your heartbeat changes once in a while. If it happens, try these methods of restoring your natural rhythm.

❖ **Take it lying down.** Whether you're walking, sweeping the floor, or cutting your grass, stop what you're doing. When you feel an attack of rapid heartbeat, sit or lie down, and relax until it's over.

❖ **Hold it!** Try holding your breath, but not for too long. This is sometimes enough to urge your heart back to its proper pace. Coughing or bearing down as if you're having a bowel movement are other methods to try.

❖ **Put on the pressure.** Pinch your nose closed and gently push against it with your breath until your ears pop. Or put your fingers over your closed eyes and press gently on your eyeballs.

❖ **Distract yourself.** Pick a sensitive area on your arm, and pinch it hard enough to really hurt.

❖ **Cool it.** Get a big bowl of ice water, hold your breath, and dunk your face. This technique is often enough of a shock to restore your normal heartbeat. A big bag of ice cubes or a towel dipped in ice water, held over your face for just a moment, may work as well. If you have angina or chest pain that gets worse in cold weather, avoid this method and try one of the others instead.

❖ **Learn massage.** If your tachycardia occurs frequently, your doctor can teach you the proper way to massage your carotid artery. This is usually an effective way to slow your rapid heartbeat, but it must be done correctly or you could hurt yourself.

The long-range plan for rapid heartbeat

Your doctor may prescribe medicine to help control your tachycardia. Here are some other ways to keep your heart on the right track.

❖ **Move it.** Regular exercise is the best way to prevent tachycardia. The healthier and stronger your heart is, the better it can maintain its own rhythm. Check with your doctor to see what kind of exercise she recommends for you.

❖ **Reduce your stress.** You probably already know that stress affects many aspects of your life. It can also add to the number of tachycardia episodes you have. Studies show that the greatest number of arrhythmias happen on Monday morning, even among retired people. Adjust your attitude or your work situation so that Monday morning isn't a big stressor for you.

❖ **Get your rest.** Working too many hours and not getting enough rest can help bring on tachycardia. Getting enough sleep (seven to eight hours for most people) may improve your efficiency at work so you can cut back on the extra hours.

❖ **If you smoke, stop.** Aside from its other health risks, smoking makes your heart beat faster and your blood vessels close up. This could make smoking a big contributor to tachycardia. Many products and programs are available to help you quit smoking. Choose one and stop.

❖ **Don't take diet pills.** The amphetamines and other stimulants in many diet pills, whether prescription or over-the-counter, will speed up your heart rate and can trigger tachycardia. A slow, steady weight loss program is a better approach to solving a weight problem.

❖ **Cut out caffeine.** You may think of your morning cup of coffee as a pleasant ritual, but it may not be the best thing for your heart. Caffeine stimulates your heart muscle to pump; too much caffeine stimulates your heart so much that it can cause palpitations and tachycardia. If rapid heartbeat is a problem for you, it's better to stay away from the caffeine in coffee, tea, and cola drinks.

❖ **Make sure of your medicine.** Tell your doctor about any drugs you are taking when she prescribes a new one. Drug interaction can cause tachycardia. For example, Seldane is a popular antihistamine that can cause serious arrhythmia and even death when it's taken with the antibiotic erythromycin or the antifungal drug Nizoral. People with liver disease may also have irregular heartbeat if they take Seldane. Since 1985, eight people have died from taking this common drug. Some ingredients in over-the-counter decongestants and other medicines may cause irregular heartbeat. Ask your doctor which ingredients in common medicines could cause problems, and read labels carefully if you have tachycardia.

❖ **Get a handle on depression.** A recent study shows that depressed people have as much as 30 percent more of a hormone called norepinephrine in their blood than people who aren't depressed. Norepinephrine raises your heart rate, so you don't want too much of it in your body. Get counseling for depression if you need to.

If you regularly have episodes of rapid heartbeat, you need your doctor's help to regulate it. But use these simple tips to gain more control over your life, your health, and the marvelous machine that is your heart.

Heartburn

A burning, heavy, uncomfortable feeling in your chest

Do you ever feel like you have a three-alarm fire burning in your chest? Fortunately, the burn usually doesn't have anything to do with your heart. The burning sensation comes from your esophagus, the tube that carries food from your mouth to your stomach.

Your stomach secretes a strong acid that is necessary for digestion. A special lining protects your stomach from the effects of this acid, but it doesn't protect your esophagus. When stomach acid backs up into your esophagus, it becomes very irritated and burns.

Although heartburn is common and rarely life-threatening, it can occasionally warn of a more serious disorder.

 ## It's time to see your doctor if you have heartburn and:

- Difficulty swallowing
- Unexplained weight loss
- Hiccups
- Cough
- Hoarseness
- Regurgitation (especially at night)

This combination of symptoms could indicate that you have a tumor of the esophagus. See your doctor immediately.

- Skin that becomes tight, thickened, and shiny (especially on your fingers and face)
- Raynaud's phenomenon (hands and feet become red, white, and blue when exposed to cold)
- Difficulty swallowing
- Joint pain and stiffness

These are some of the symptoms of scleroderma, a rare but potentially fatal disease in which your immune system attacks its own tissues. In mild cases, it affects only your skin, but severe cases involve other organs and tissues, including your heart, lungs, kidneys, gastrointestinal tract, and joints. In a few rare cases, scleroderma can rapidly lead to death from heart, respiratory, or kidney failure.

How to tell heartburn from a heart attack

Heartburn can sometimes feel like a heart attack, but, in most cases, if you're having a heart attack, you'll also have other symptoms. For example:

❖ Pain that spreads to your shoulders, arms, neck, or jaw

❖ Lightheadedness, fainting

❖ Sweating

❖ Nausea

❖ Shortness of breath

If you think you are having a heart attack, get help immediately.

- **Loss of appetite**
- **Nausea, vomiting**
- **Stomach pain, tenderness, or cramping, often worsened by eating**

If you have these symptoms, you may have gastritis, an inflammation of the lining of your stomach. If symptoms are caused by a virus or a food you've eaten, they will normally disappear within two to three days. If they don't, see your doctor. (See also *Appetite loss* chapter.)

- **Angina-like chest pain**
- **Difficulty swallowing**
- **Acid-tasting stomach contents sometimes rise into mouth when belching**
- **Chronic cough**

If you have these symptoms, especially if they get worse at night, you may have gastroesophageal reflux disease (GERD). In this condition, stomach acid backs up into your esophagus and irritates the lining, causing an uncomfortable burning sensation. If you suffer from GERD for a long period of time, your esophagus can suffer severe damage, and it can increase your risk of cancer. Don't just ignore these symptoms. See your doctor.

Immediate help for gastroesophageal reflux disease

After eating a heavy, satisfying meal, all you want to do is lie down and take it easy. "Resting helps digestion," your grandmother used to say, but lying down after a meal causes painful burning in your chest. To relieve the discomfort, you'll probably reach for an antacid. Antacids provide quick, temporary relief. They neutralize the stomach acid that can splash back into your esophagus and set your chest on fire.

Liquid antacids tend to work better than tablets. Keep your liquid in the refrigerator. A cold antacid tastes better, which makes it easier to swallow. Antacids don't do any good if you take them with meals, so take them after meals or just before bedtime.

Choosing an antacid can be confusing. Consider the following types:

❖ **Sodium bicarbonates.** These are the kind that go plop plop, fizz fizz (or just fizz fizz). Plain old baking

---

Hiatal hernia and heartburn

A hiatal hernia occurs when part of your stomach moves up into your chest through an opening in your diaphragm. Some doctors think a hiatal hernia can cause your esophageal valve to weaken, allowing stomach acid to leak into your esophagus.

No one seems to know what causes hiatal hernias, but they can be made worse by coughing, straining, strenuous abdominal exercises, obesity, pregnancy, or vomiting.

Hiatal hernias usually don't require treatment, but if the hernia is in danger of becoming twisted or is causing severe GERD, surgery may be required.

soda is sodium bicarbonate, and so is Alka Seltzer. They act very quickly and are not expensive, but because they contain lots of sodium, they can be harmful if you use them too often. If you are on a low-salt diet, or if you have high blood pressure, don't use this kind of antacid.

❖ **Calcium carbonates.** These include the candy-flavored antacids like Tums and Rolaids. They also work well for most people, but they contain a lot of calcium, which can actually cause you to produce more acid. If used too often, they may cause kidney stones.

❖ **Magnesium and aluminum.** These may be the safest kind to use over a long period of time. Magnesium alone can cause diarrhea, so most products combine magnesium and aluminum. These include brands like Maalox, Gaviscon, and Mylanta. Although these don't contain too much calcium or sodium, they still shouldn't be used if you have severe kidney disease.

The long-range plan for gastroesophageal reflux disease

While antacids may quench the fire of heartburn temporarily, they can cause side effects if used regularly. The best way to douse the fire is to practice prevention. Your esophagus is protected from acid splash-back by a valve called the lower esophageal sphincter or LES, but sometimes your LES goes to sleep on the job. It relaxes and allows stomach contents to sneak past it into your unprotected esophagus. Anything that may put pressure on this valve or cause it to relax may set you up to get burned by heartburn.

Here are some things you can do to keep your lower esophageal sphincter in good shape:

❖ **Kick the habit.** A cigarette is a double-edged sword as far as GERD is concerned. The smoke causes a temporary reduction in the strength of the esophageal valve, and the nicotine increases your production of stomach acid. Remember, the next time you light up, you may also be lighting a painful fire in your chest.

❖ **Avoid food triggers.** Certain foods are more likely to trigger an attack of heartburn, probably because they cause your LES to relax. Although different people have different triggers, some of the more common ones include chocolate, peppermint, spearmint, caffeine, tomatoes, citrus juices, and spicy foods. You can keep a food diary to help you identify the foods that give you heartburn.

❖ **Eat small meals.** Large meals seem to bring on heartburn more than light meals. You may be better off eating six small meals throughout the day instead of eating three large meals.

❖ **Stand up straight.** You knew there was a reason your mother chastised you for your posture. Bending or stooping after meals can force food and stomach acid into your esophagus, setting off the fire of heartburn. For the same reason, you should avoid eating right before going to bed.

❖ **Keep it slim.** Excess weight may increase pressure in your abdominal area, which can make food more likely to back up into your esophagus.

❖ **Let it all hang out.** Though you may be tempted to tuck those excess pounds into a girdle or tight-fitting jeans, you may pay a price for your vanity. Just like that extra fat, the pressure from tight clothing can force food upward. Loosen your belt a notch or two and wear loose, comfortable clothing.

❖ **Raise your head.** You should raise the head of your bed so your head is higher than your stomach. Most heartburn occurs at night, while you are lying down. If you put a 6-inch block under the head of your bed, or under your box spring, you will have the force of gravity on your side. Stomach acid will be much less likely to back up into your esophagus, and you can get a good night's sleep.

❖ **Try to remain regular.** Straining to have a bowel movement can make your reflux worse. (See the *Constipation* chapter for advice on remaining regular.) Exercises like sit-ups and leg lifts may also cause additional strain.

❖ **Avoid aspirin and alcohol.** Alcohol and aspirin can aggravate your reflux, so limit your intake of alcohol and use a pain reliever containing acetaminophen, like Tylenol, instead of aspirin.

❖ **Check your medicine cabinet.** Many prescription drugs can cause heartburn. Some of the most common include Bentyl and Librax, which are used to treat intestinal spasms, and Inderal, Lopressor, Cardizem, Calan, and Verapamil, which are used to treat high blood pressure and angina. Ask your doctor or pharmacist if your heartburn could be caused by the medicine you are taking.

Treatment for persistent heartburn

If you have an occasional flare-up of heartburn, you probably reach for an antacid for quick relief, but did you know long-term use of antacids may cause side effects?

Don't despair. New, over-the-counter medicine is available to treat acid reflux. The first to be introduced was Tagamet (cimetidine), and it was followed by Zantac (ranitidine), Pepcid (famotidine), and Axid (nizatidine). These drugs decrease the amount of acid your stomach produces. You take them once or twice a day, instead of constantly chewing an antacid tablet. If all else fails, see your doctor. He can prescribe medicine that will extinguish the fire.

Hip pain

Discomfort in the joint between the pelvis and the thigh

Your hip is a strong, ball-and-socket joint connecting the long bone of your thigh to your pelvis. Without its unique design, you wouldn't be able to twist and bend, cross your legs, or curl up in an easy chair.

Like all your joints, the hip receives its fair share of use and abuse, so it isn't any wonder that things go wrong. Even though athletes commonly complain of hip pain, you don't have to be a gymnast, dancer, or even a runner to feel an occasional ache. Simply straining the long muscle down the outside of your thigh can make your hip area hurt. You could even have pain somewhere else, such as your feet, buttocks, or ankles, and still feel it in your hip. After all, everything is connected in some way to everything else.

You may have been born with one leg longer than the other — and suffer hip pain as a result. Just a few centimeters can be enough to affect how you stand and walk. Most people never realize they have this problem; they simply adjust to the condition. Shoe inserts are an easy way to correct it.

If you have hip pain for more than two weeks, it could mean something serious.

⚕ It's time to see your doctor if you have hip pain and:

- Pain within the bones of the hip, pelvis, and femur that is worse at night
- Swelling of the hip joint
- A fracture of the hip without cause

With these symptoms, it is possible you have a malignant growth in your hip, or bone cancer. The most common type is secondary bone cancer, which spreads from the breast, lung, prostate, thyroid, or kidney to the bones.

- Morning joint stiffness
- Limited movement and dexterity

This could mean osteoarthritis, a condition where the cartilage in your joints gradually breaks down.

207

Usually, you will feel an aching pain when you move or put weight on your joints. (See also *Knee pain* chapter.)

- **Swelling and redness in the hip**
- **Low fever**
- **General ill-feeling**
- **Severe morning stiffness that can last for hours**

Hip fracture

If you fracture your hip, you're actually breaking the top of your femur, the long bone of your thigh. Each year, about 200,000 adults over the age of 65 suffer such a break, usually because of a fall. If you have osteoporosis, you're at especially high risk because your bones are so brittle.

Since everyone loses muscle tone and strength as they age, it is especially important to get a lot of calcium in your system, stay strong and active, and protect yourself against falls.

If you fall down and have the following symptoms, you may have a fractured hip. See your doctor right away.

- Severe pain while trying to walk

- Swelling and bruising

- Unnatural shape of the hip area

- Injured leg is shorter

- Knee pain instead of hip pain

In this case, you may have no choice but surgery. It's usually the only treatment for a hip fracture. Your bone pieces will be reattached and secured with pins or screws. By the day after surgery, you should be able to walk around with help. You'll probably need a walker or cane for several weeks, but with the appropriate physical therapy, you should see a full recovery.

These symptoms may indicate the onset of rheumatoid arthritis, a disease that inflames the joints.
Resting may not bring you relief from the pain.

- Pain on one side of your body, in your buttock and
  leg
- Stiffness in your lower back
- Muscle spasms beside your spine
- Increased pain when bending, straining, coughing,
  or sneezing

The sciatic nerve is the largest nerve running from
the lower back down each leg. When this nerve is
irritated by back problems, you can have pain all
the way from your lower back to your toes. This is
called sciatica. It can be caused by injury, arthritis,
or infection.

- Recent injury
- Swelling
- Restricted movement of your hip

If you have injured your hip and damaged the ligaments holding the bones together, you may have
dislocated the joint. This is a serious injury, and
your doctor should decide appropriate action.

- Redness and swelling in your hip joint
- Severe pain that usually occurs at night

Gout is a form of acute arthritis marked by inflammation of the joints. It is caused by too much uric
acid in the blood, which forms crystals in the
joints. Attacks usually last about a week.

- Swollen hip joint with muscle stiffness
- Headaches
- Anxiety or depression
- Fatigue
- Irritable bowel syndrome or bladder problems

These symptoms, along with muscle pain in your
neck and shoulders, could be caused by fibromyalgia.
This is a puzzling condition that can be mistaken

for many other more serious diseases. You need to see a specialist for an accurate diagnosis.

- **Recurring backache or sudden back pain after bending or lifting**
- **Curved spine, often with humps**
- **Loss of several inches in height**
- **Easily fractured bone, usually your hip or arm**

Osteoporosis is a gradual break down of your bones due to a loss of calcium and phosphate salts. Your bones lose density, become brittle, and are easily fractured.

- **Heat, redness, and swelling**
- **Any type of broken skin near your hip**

These are signs of an infection. See your doctor.

- **Inflammation of the hip joint**
- **Restricted movement of your hip**
- **Hip pain when crossing your legs**
- **Injury or strain to the hip within a week of symp-toms**

Bursae are small, fluid-filled sacs that act as cushions between the working parts of your joints. When a joint is injured or strained, these bursae can become inflamed. This is called bursitis.

Immediate help for bursitis

Your joints are constantly moving. That is the nature of their job. But because a joint is made up of hard bones and relatively soft tendons, the friction between them could cause some real damage if nature didn't give you some protection — namely, the bursa.

Bursitis occurs when this bursa swells up, usually in the shoulder, elbow, hip socket, kneecap, or ankle joint. You may have injured yourself recently, or perhaps it's those years of dedicated running that abused your joints and set off your bursitis. Rheumatoid arthritis or gout can cause this condition as well.

Your doctor may prescribe a strong anti-inflammatory drug to bring down the swelling, give you an injection of corticosteroids, or remove the fluid in the bursa to reduce swelling. Usually, recent cases of bursitis can be cured within a week. To help speed your recovery:

❖ **Rest.** Since overuse probably had something to do with your attack of bursitis, resting the joint will go a long way toward fixing it. A few days of being a couch potato will give the swollen bursa a chance to heal.

❖ **Then get off the couch.** Rest is good for a few days, but don't get used to it, or your joints will stiffen up. Stand up, change positions, walk around — just get moving.

❖ **Cool it down.** If you are experiencing intense pain, try an ice pack or gel-filled cold pack. Never apply ice directly to your skin. You may give yourself a case of frostbite and damage your tissues.

❖ **Relieve the pain.** Take aspirin or ibuprofen to relieve pain and bring down the swelling. Acetaminophen (Tylenol) won't help the swelling, but many people combine it with the other two. Check with your doctor first.

❖ **Sit up straight.** You probably thought no one but your mother would say that to you, but experts agree that good posture is better for your joints. So, shoulders back, head up, back straight, and ... smile.

❖ **Do's and don'ts.** Toss the high heels to the back of the closet. You need comfortable, cushioned shoes that support your leg and place less stress on your joints. Avoid climbing stairs, if possible, and opt for the short walk around the block rather than the trailblazing hike.

The long-range plan for bursitis

Bursitis has no cure, but with common-sense treatment, you can live a normal, relatively pain-free life.

❖ **Assess your activities.** Did you overdo it a bit during your last golf game? Are there other activities that set your bursitis off? Think about what you do regularly that makes you uncomfortable. It may be time to adjust your lifestyle. Yoga, walking, swimming, and gardening are all excellent activities that will gently work and stretch your body.

❖ **Pain IS no gain.** Forget the drill sergeant routine. It shouldn't hurt. When it does, stop. Normal, slow joint movement is good therapy for bursitis and will gradually make your hip more flexible and movable.

❖ **Check your weight.** If you are carrying extra pounds, you're placing extra stress on your hips and other joints. Consult your doctor and begin a sensible weight-loss program.

Impotence

Inability to achieve or maintain an erection
Erections are too painful, weak, or brief for intercourse
Decrease in size or rigidity of erection
Loss of body hair

The very indignity of impotence makes this problem difficult for many men to talk about. Even though impotence is not a top topic for conversation, it's not because so few men suffer from this problem. Actually, about 30 million American men struggle with chronic impotence. That means about three out of every eight men have to deal with some form of this problem.

Before you panic over the apparent inability of your penis to perform, check your lifestyle for clues. How's your stress level? Too much stress will sap even the most ardent man's sexual energy. What's your diet like? If you aren't eating a balanced diet or taking a multivitamin, you may be deficient in zinc, which can contribute to the development of impotence in some men.

Had surgery or an accident lately? Surgery of the bladder, colon, prostate, or rectum may cause impotence if any blood vessels or nerve paths that help engineer an erection get damaged while you're under the knife. If you've had any pelvic or groin injury, such as falling on the crossbar of a bike, it may have damaged the blood flow to your penis, resulting in impotence. Other activities where you may suffer such groin or pelvic injuries include gymnastics, horseback riding, and water sports. Injuries to the spinal cord or brain may also cause impotence.

In addition, alcohol and cigarette addictions, a breakdown in communication with your partner, or finding your partner unattractive can all dampen desire. An illness may also temporarily affect your sexual abilities. And once you become anxious about your impotence, it can turn from an occasional occurrence into a chronic complaint.

The good news is almost all cases of impotence can be treated successfully. In fact, according to the Impotence Resource Center, "Impotence is the most untreated, treatable medical disorder in the world." Although this disorder can be treated successfully 95 percent of the time, only 5 percent of people with this problem actually receive treatment. Personal embarrassment and lack of knowledge prevent many men from seeking the medical help they need.

Your first step should be to see a urologist, a doctor who deals with problems of the urogenital tract, to determine if a medical problem is causing your impotence. In 80 percent of the cases of impotence, the root of the problem is a medical disorder, such as vascular disease, diabetes, or leaking veins. For men over 40, clogged arteries and leaky veins are the most common cause. Diabetes can also interfere with proper blood flow to the penis.

If your doctor can't diagnose a definite medical problem, see a psychologist. A physical problem can actually lead to a psychological disorder. Once your mind sees you fail a couple of times, your fear of failure tends to reinforce your problem.

 It's time to see your doctor if you have impotence and:

  Excessive thirst

- Increased appetite
- Frequent urination
- Unexplained weight loss
- Frequent infections
- Fatigue

You may have diabetes. Since you will need insulin to control this disorder, you should schedule an appointment with your doctor as soon as possible. (See also *Weight changes, unexplained* chapter.)

- Poor muscle coordination, clumsiness, stiffness
- Difficulty speaking
- Blurred or double vision
- Problems remembering recent events

These symptoms may indicate a disorder of your nervous system, such as multiple sclerosis, Alzheimer's, or Parkinson's disease. See your doctor immediately. (See also *Forgetfulness* chapter.)

- Lack of energy
- Difficulty handling cold or stress
- Loss of appetite, nausea
- Frequent headaches

Your symptoms suggest an underactive pituitary gland. See your doctor immediately. This disorder can be fatal if not treated promptly.

- Feel cold all the time
- Decreased sweating
- Decreased appetite
- Chest pain
- Weight gain
- Feel sleepy or have trouble sleeping
- Feel depressed or have trouble remembering things

These symptoms might indicate that you have hypothyroidism, or an underactive thyroid. Although hypothyroidism is generally easy to treat with thyroid-replacement hormones, it can cause life-threatening complications in rare cases, so it is important to see your doctor. (See also *Weight changes, unexplained* chapter.)

- Unusual discharge from penis
- Blisters or sores on penis, may or may not be itchy or painful
- Swollen lymph nodes

If you have any one of these symptoms, you may be suffering from a sexually transmitted disease. See your doctor immediately for treatment.

- Tiredness, weakness
- Yellow eyes and skin
- Loss of appetite, nausea
- Palms of hands appear very red

You may have cirrhosis of the liver. See your doctor immediately.

- Boredom, down mood
- Lack of energy
- Difficulty sleeping or sleeping too much
- Loss of appetite or overeating
- No interest in doing things you used to enjoy
- Problems concentrating or making decisions
- Feeling useless
- Feel irritable, restless, withdrawn
- Excessive guilt feelings for no real cause
- Headaches or chest pains that don't have any physical cause

These symptoms suggest you may be suffering from depression. If self-help methods don't help or you feel suicidal, see a doctor immediately. (See also *Depression* chapter.)

- Feel nervous, edgy, and worried
- Rapid, pounding heartbeat
- Tight or squeezing sensation in the chest
- Difficulty breathing, shortness of breath
- Overwhelming fears, poor memory and concentration
- Blurred vision or eyelid twitching
- Regular backaches, headaches, or neck aches

Any combination of these symptoms may mean you are suffering from severe anxiety or panic disorder.

Stress, guilt, alcohol, drugs, or working too hard can cause anxiety and lead to chest pain. (See also *Anxiety* chapter.)

- Fatigue
- Depression
- Irritability

Your symptoms suggest you may be suffering from hypogonadism, sometimes called male menopause, caused by a lack of testosterone. This disorder may be triggered by stress, obesity, alcoholism, surgery, or certain drugs. Your doctor can do a simple blood test to see if you have hypogonadism. If the test shows you do have a deficiency, testosterone replacement therapy will soon have you feeling like your old self again.

- Leg cramps
- Chest pain
- Headache
- Dizziness

You may have atherosclerosis, a condition in which fat builds up on your artery walls and restricts blood flow. More commonly known as "hardening of the arteries," atherosclerosis is a major cause of fatal heart disease and stroke in the U.S.

Immediate help for atherosclerosis

If your doctor just revealed that your impotence is a side effect of atherosclerosis, consider yourself lucky. You could have been dead. That's the only warning of clogged arteries some folks ever get.

Doubtless you don't consider your impotence an immense stroke of luck, but it may not be as bad as it seems either. Now that you know what's causing your problem, you can prevent the atherosclerosis from getting worse. Some doctors even suggest you may be able to reverse the process — that is, actually clear out the arteries that are clogged.

216

That may mean even more to your health than recovering your sexual abilities since atherosclerosis is responsible for a number of other disorders, including heart disease, stroke, kidney failure, senility, and even gangrene.

The six steps below will help get your health, and your sex life, back on track.

- ❖ **Stop smoking.** Despite what television shows and slick magazine ads might make you believe, smoking isn't sexy. In fact, it's not only a nasty habit, it can make your sex life stink. Smoking contributes to blockages in the arteries that lead to the penis. Without adequate blood flow, your penis can't maintain an erection.

- ❖ **Control your cholesterol.** Men with total cholesterol higher than 240 mg/dl are twice as likely to have trouble achieving or maintaining an erection than men whose cholesterol levels are below 180 mg/dl. Men who have low levels of HDL, the good cholesterol, are also twice as likely to suffer from impotence. Limit cholesterol you eat to less than 300 mg per day. An easy way to cut cholesterol is to limit your intake of butter, cheese, eggs, and meats, especially red meat.

- ❖ **Keep a cap on blood pressure.** High blood pressure forces your heart to work harder to move blood through your body. The extra effort can damage your arteries and pave the way for atherosclerosis. The healthiest blood pressure is 120 over 80 or less. High blood pressure is defined as 140 or more over 90 or more. Have your blood pressure checked regularly so you'll know where you stand. If you'd like to see those numbers drop a little, eat a low-fat, low-calorie, low-salt diet. Walking regularly will help you drop any excess pounds you're carrying, which also lowers blood pressure.

- ❖ **Manage your stress.** Chronic stress causes your noradrenaline and adrenaline hormone levels to remain high. This leads to excessive production of cortisol and other steroids, which causes blockages in your arteries to build up faster. Arteries partially clogged by fat tend to constrict more than normal arteries in response to stress, which further limits your already reduced blood flow. See Stress chapter for suggestions on handling stress.

❖ **Socialize.** Studies show that people with social ties and connections to other people have fewer artery blockages than people who don't have these connections.

❖ **Perk up your penis with pelvic exercises.** Although some doctors say pelvic muscles don't have any influence on blood flow to the penis, a new study suggests otherwise. Recently, a team of Belgian urologists treated 150 men who suffered from impotence. Some men had operations and others did special pelvic muscle exercises called Kegels. One year after treatment, 58 percent of the men who performed the Kegel exercises were completely cured or were so satisfied with their improvement that they did not opt for surgery. Try Kegels for yourself. It certainly can't hurt, and it may help.

How to do Kegel exercises

1. Identify the pelvic muscles that need exercising. You can do this by stopping and starting the flow of urine several times when using the bathroom.
2. Tighten the muscles a little at a time. Contract muscles slowly, hold for a count of 10, and relax the muscles slowly.
3. Repeat these exercises for the anal pelvic muscles. To find these muscles, imagine you're trying to hold back a bowel movement, without tensing your leg, stomach, or buttock muscles.
4. Practice tightening all pelvic muscles together, moving from back to front.
5. Start with five repetitions of each exercise three to five times a day. Gradually work up to 20 or 30 repetitions at once.

The long-range plan for atherosclerosis

When it comes to preventing and even reversing atherosclerosis, most of the suggestions center around controlling your cholesterol. That's because cholesterol

Sexual energy sapped by drugs

If you hope to have a satisfying sex life, it's important to avoid romance-robbing drugs.

More than 200 different prescription drugs can cause impotence. Side effects can appear after only a few weeks or develop after you've been taking a drug for years.

First on the list are blood pressure drugs and diuretics. Tranquilizers and other psychiatric drugs, antihistamines, antidepressants, beta blockers, decongestants, and many over-the counter remedies, like cold medicines, can also cause problems. Drinking alcohol, smoking, or using illegal drugs, such as cocaine and marijuana, can also cause impotence.

Other drugs that can cause problems include:

❖ Anti-ulcer drugs

❖ Hormones, including birth control pills

❖ Reserpine

❖ Digitalis

❖ Skeletal muscle relaxants

Your problem may be caused either by a reaction to the drug or as a drug side effect. If you're using a nonprescription drug you think may be contributing to your problem, stop taking it or switch to something else.

However, if you suspect a prescription drug is interfering with your love life, never stop taking it or switch medicine without talking to your doctor. Such a decision can be deadly. Your doctor can help you find a safe alternative. And the next time you get a new prescription, ask about the effects it could have on your sex life.

makes up the main part of the plaque that sticks to blood vessel walls and clogs arteries.

Cholesterol combines with two forms of lipoproteins to travel in your body: high-density lipoprotein (HDL) and low-density lipoprotein (LDL). Both contain fat and protein, but LDL is mostly fat, while HDL is mostly protein.

They also perform different functions in your body. HDL takes excess fat and cholesterol from tissues to the liver to be dismantled. LDL carries fat and cholesterol to your body's tissues.

High levels of LDL forecast a high risk of heart disease, while high levels of HDL indicate a low risk. Here are some suggestions to help ensure your HDL level stays high and your LDL level stays low:

❖ **Learn to love low-fat.** Dr. Dean Ornish, author of *Dr. Dean Ornish's Program for Reversing Heart Disease*, recommends that no more than 10 percent of your calories come from fat. Even though this diet may sound difficult, it's really very simple. Just center your meals around fruits, vegetables, grains, legumes (such as beans and peas), and soybean products. Stay away from high-fat vegetarian foods like avocados, olives, coconut, nuts, and seeds. You should also avoid all animal products with the exception of egg whites and 1 cup of nonfat yogurt or milk a day. Limit alcohol to 2 ounces per day or less and avoid caffeine, which can provoke stress.

❖ **Fill up on fiber.** Fiber helps bind up cholesterol in your intestines, preventing it from being absorbed and clogging your arteries. You need at least 30 grams of fiber a day. Grains, fruits, and vegetables are all good sources. Dr. Mary Dan Eades, author of *The Doctor's Complete Guide to Vitamins and Minerals*, recommends 50 or more grams a day. She suggests supplementing the fiber in your diet with a vegetable fiber bulking powder such as Metamucil or Citrucel. Add more fiber to your diet gradually or you're likely to suffer from bloating, cramping, and gas.

❖ **Take vitamin E to make life easier on your arteries.** A recent study reported that men who took a supplement of 100 IU (international units) of vitamin E daily developed significantly less artery blockage than men who took less than 100 IU.

❖ **Fight your thirst with fruit juice.** Researchers have discovered that grape juice contains flavonoids that offer powerful antioxidant protection, which helps keep cholesterol from damaging your artery walls. Grapefruit juice can also lower the level of cholesterol in your blood and improves the ratio of good cholesterol to bad. Grapefruit juice may also help you get rid of the fatty buildup, called plaque, in your arteries that can cause blockages.

❖ **Eat more garlic.** Eating as little as a half of clove of garlic a day reduces cholesterol an average of 9 percent, according to researchers at New York's Medical College. It also lowers blood pressure and prevents the bad LDL cholesterol from being oxidized, which damages arteries. Since lower cholesterol means lower risk of fat buildup on your artery walls, a little garlic every day could do your body good.

❖ **Limit foods that make your body produce insulin.** These include refined starches and sugars, such as white flour, highly milled cornmeal, table sugar, corn syrup, molasses, and any products made using these items. High insulin levels stimulate your body to make more cholesterol — just what you don't want.

❖ **Get moving.** Exercise is an excellent way to raise your HDL level. Jogging or walking briskly for 30 minutes three to five times a week will significantly raise your HDLs.

❖ **Take time for tea.** Green tea, and possibly black tea, may lower your cholesterol and improve your HDL to LDL ratio.

❖ **Make sure you get enough folic acid.** Homocysteine, one of the amino acids used to make protein, may also promote hardening of the arteries. Folic acid turns homocysteine into the amino acid methionine, which does not have this effect. Your best bet is to look for a B-complex supplement that supplies the RDA for folic acid, which is 400 micrograms (mcg), and also includes other B vitamins. The B vitamins work best together.

❖ **Feel vibrant with vitamin C.** A recent study revealed that people who took more than 60 milligrams (mg) of vitamin C a day, the recommended dietary allowance, had the highest HDL levels.

❖ **Crunch atherosclerosis with calcium.** A calcium carbonate supplement lowered total cholesterol 4 percent and raised good HDL cholesterol 4 percent in a group of 56 people who took 400 mg of calcium three times a day.

❖ **Zap the zinc.** If you have a problem with cholesterol, don't take zinc supplements. Zinc interferes with your body's absorption of copper, which can lower good HDL and raise bad LDL. When purchasing a multivitamin, look for one that contains the least amount of zinc.

Incontinence

Inability to control the bladder and/or bowel

Everyone likes to be in control of his life, whether it involves choosing a job, where to go on vacation, or when to walk the dog. Each decision becomes a tiny statement of control.

That is why losing control of basic body functions may seem like a loss of power or independence. But that doesn't have to be the case. Remember, there are physical reasons for your incontinence. Most of them require professional attention.

It's time to see your doctor if you have incontinence and:

- Headache
- Blurred or double vision
- Dizziness and confusion
- Vomiting
- Fever
- Inability to speak
- Inability to move one side of your body

You suffer brain damage when your blood and oxygen supply is reduced or cut off to a portion of your brain. This is a stroke — a medical emergency. You may have different symptoms depending on how severe the stroke is and which artery it affects. Get help immediately. (See also *Slurred speech* chapter.)

- Memory loss
- Disorientation/confusion
- Anxiety
- Insomnia
- Lack of concentration
- Difficulty communicating and completing tasks
- Gradual changes in personality and mental abilities

These are just a few symptoms of Alzheimer's disease, a condition where your brain function gradually breaks down. Many treatable diseases, including depression, have the same symptoms as Alzheimer's, so get a thorough medical exam if you suspect this problem. (See also *Forgetfulness* chapter.)

- Muscle weakness, clumsiness, stiffness
- Blurred or double vision
- Difficulty speaking
- Impotence
- Fatigue
- Numbness or tingling

This combination of symptoms could mean you have multiple sclerosis, a disorder of your nervous system. It usually begins in early adulthood.

- Unusual discharge from penis (men)
- Blisters or sores on penis that may or may not be itchy or painful (men)
- Genital itching (women)
- Vaginal discharge (women)
- Swollen lymph nodes
- Painful urination

If you have any one of these symptoms, you may be suffering from a sexually transmitted disease. See your doctor immediately for treatment.

- A sudden sharp pain down the back of your leg
- Numbness or tingling in an arm or leg
- Back pain

These symptoms could indicate pressure or damage to your spine from a ruptured disk. (See also **Back pain** chapter.)

(For men only)
- A frequent and urgent need to urinate, but difficulty beginning
- A weak stream of urine that sometimes dribbles
- Inability to empty the bladder completely

The prostate is a gland that lies under the bladder and surrounds the urethra. Most men over 50 will experience some enlargement of this gland, known as benign prostatic hyperplasia, perhaps due to hormonal changes. If the overgrowth is severe enough, it will interfere with the flow of urine.

- Inability to have a normal bowel movement
- Feeling of constipation, but involuntary diarrhea
- Abdominal pain or cramping (sometimes)

You could be suffering from a severe case of constipation, called fecal impaction. This condition is usually curable, but you and your doctor need to determine what caused the impaction to prevent it from recurring. (See also *Constipation* chapter.)

> Involuntary loss of urine when coughing, sneezing, laughing, or during physical activity

If you suffer this common problem, you're a victim of stress incontinence.

Immediate help for stress incontinence

Stress incontinence may affect more than 10 million Americans, most of them women over 50, but their doctors will never know. People seem to think incontinence is a natural part of aging. Couple that with the humiliation they feel over "leaking," and you have what many experts call the "silent epidemic."

Your body changes a great deal as you age, but that alone will not lead to stress urinary incontinence (SUI). You're more likely to develop SUI from certain drugs, diseases, and conditions. Even if you find it embarrassing, you must discuss your symptoms with your doctor, so she can properly diagnosis your problem. In the meantime, here are some things you can do to regain control over this part of your life.

❖ **Check your menu.** Many foods and drinks affect your ability to hold urine. Watch your intake of coffee, tea, carbonated drinks, citrus fruits, tomatoes, chocolate, sugar, honey, spicy foods, and milk products. Perhaps one or more of these are adding to the problem.

❖ **Keep drinking.** Don't try to control your incontinence by drinking less. It is still important to keep your body well-hydrated. Experts recommend six to eight glasses of water each day.

❖ **Take care of your skin.** If your incontinence continues, the skin in that area may become irritated and possibly infected. Keep your skin clean and dry, using mild soap, warm water, and soft towels. Ask your pharmacist about an appropriate cream or ointment to protect your skin as well.

Drugs that cause incontinence

❖ Antipsychotic agents

❖ Antihistamines

❖ Antidepressants

❖ Decongestants

❖ Diuretics

❖ Antihypertensives

❖ Sedative-hypnotics

The long-range plan for stress incontinence

You can wear an absorbent product to give you some peace of mind and let you participate in activities you enjoy. But you can also take a more active part in controlling your incontinence. It may take some time and effort, and you may have to change your lifestyle somewhat, but it also could help you avoid surgery. Discuss all options with your doctor, but try these self-help tips first.

❖ **Train your bladder.** By going to the bathroom on a strict schedule, you teach your bladder to hold more urine, and avoid waiting too long to visit the bathroom. You should keep a chart or diary, and begin by going to the toilet every 30 minutes. Gradually increase the time to every two to three hours.

❖ **Work out.** Kegel exercises are a great way to strengthen the muscles that control your urine flow. Sit comfortably with your legs uncrossed and your abdominal, thigh, and buttocks muscles relaxed. Then pretend you are trying to stop urinating. The muscles that you tighten are called pubococcygeus muscles. Keep them tense for about 10 seconds, then relax. Repeat this tensing and relaxing 10 times, three times a day. Be patient. You may not see improvement for at least six to eight weeks, and you may have to make the exercises part of your daily routine. If you want to check to be sure you are doing them right, you can buy something called vaginal cones. Insert one of the weighted plastic cones into your vagina, and tighten the muscles to hold the cone in place. If you are doing the Kegels correctly, the cone will not fall out. Remember to tighten these muscles before you cough, sneeze, or lift a heavy object to help control any leaking. Soon, you may not even have to think about it.

❖ **Buy into biofeedback.** A professional can train you in this technique to help you become more aware of how your body works. This will help you gain more control over your bladder.

❖ **Stay active.** Keep as regular an exercise program as possible. This will not only contribute to your overall health, but will keep your bowel movements regular. Constipation can affect incontinence.

❖ **Stop smoking.** Tobacco smoke affects your bladder and urethra. So do conditions associated with cigarettes, such as asthma and circulatory diseases. And that hacking smoker's cough places a lot of stress on your bladder, which can lead to leakage. It's never too late to quit. Ask your doctor for help.

Insomnia

The inability to fall asleep or stay asleep

Do you lie awake at night, unable to drift off for hours, only to require three different alarm clocks to wake you up in the morning? If so, you're probably not functioning very well during the day. Insomnia may not be a life-threatening illness like cancer, but the daytime drowsiness that it causes can threaten your job and your happiness. And if it makes you fall asleep behind the wheel, it can indirectly threaten not only your life, but others as well.

 ## It's time to see your doctor if you have insomnia and:

- Shortness of breath or difficulty breathing, especially when lying down
- Cough
- Irregular or rapid heartbeat
- Weakness, fatigue, or faintness
- Swollen stomach, legs, and ankles
- Breathing difficulty

Together, these symptoms may indicate congestive heart failure, which is usually a complication of other illnesses such as heart or lung disease.

- Loud, long, and frequent snoring
- Drowsiness
- Weight problems
- Early morning headaches
- Nighttime breathing difficulties
- Sexual dysfunction

These symptoms indicate you may suffer from sleep apnea. (See also *Drowsiness* chapter.)

- Drowsiness/frequent periods of sudden sleep
- Attacks of waking paralysis set off by strong emotions
- Intense dreams just after falling asleep or just before waking
- Brief, sudden loss of muscle control, sometimes causing collapse
- Lapse of recent memory, even in the middle of an activity
- Frequent nighttime awakenings
- Blurred vision

Narcolepsy is a rare sleeping disorder that can be easily misdiagnosed, but dream-like hallucinations and paralysis help to identify this condition. If you are diagnosed with narcolepsy, protect yourself from those sudden sleep attacks by not driving long distances or working with dangerous machinery.

* Decreased appetite, sweating, and tolerance for cold
* Chest pain
* Weight gain or extreme thinness
* Mental problems like depression or poor memory

These symptoms may mean you have hypothyroidism, or an underactive thyroid. Although hypothyroidism is generally easy to treat with thyroid replacement drugs, it can cause life-threatening complications in rare cases, so it is important to see your doctor. (See also *Weight changes, unexplained* chapter.)

Immediate help for insomnia

Everyone can deal with an occasional sleepless night. You may not be your usual bubbly self the following day, but you know your insomnia is just a passing phase. Temporary insomnia is usually caused by stress. If you're moving, taking a new job, getting married or perhaps divorced, you'll probably have trouble sleeping for a few nights. But if your insomnia persists, it may start interfering with your job, your family time, and your social life.

Insomnia usually falls into one of two categories. If you can't fall asleep, you have what is known as sleep-onset insomnia. If you fall asleep easily, but wake up every two hours, or at 4 a.m. every day, you have maintenance insomnia. Either way, you're not getting enough sleep, and you want help.

When you're desperately counting sheep, and you still can't fall asleep, you may be tempted to reach into your medicine cabinet for help. However, sleeping pills can be addictive, and may make your insomnia worse in the long run. See your doctor to make sure your insomnia isn't caused by a medical problem. Then, try some of the self-help suggestions below before you reach for an over-the-counter solution.

Drugs that cause insomnia

You're exhausted from tossing and turning, and you've tried every trick you know to help you nod off, but nothing works. You're so frustrated, you're ready to rummage through your medicine cabinet for sleeping pills. Before you dig them out, however, take a look at the other bottles in your medicine cabinet. One of them may hold the answer to your sleepless nights. Several types of drugs can cause insomnia as a side effect. Some of the common ones are:

❖ Antihypertensives

❖ Antineoplastics

❖ Beta-blockers

❖ Corticosteroids

❖ Decongestants

❖ Diuretics

❖ Levodopa

❖ Oral contraceptives

❖ Phenytoin (Dilantin)

❖ Selective serotonin reuptake inhibitors and protriptyline (Vivactil)

❖ Stimulants

❖ Theophylline

❖ Thyroid hormone

Alcohol and caffeine sometimes are ingredients in over-the-counter medicines, so you don't have to drink coffee or wine to get their eye-opening effects. Read the labels on all medicines carefully, and if you think your medicine may be causing your insomnia, ask your doctor if you can change medicines or lower your dosage.

❖ **Wind down slowly.** You're lying in bed unable to sleep, the day's events going round and round in your head. Try to head off this problem by taking about 30 minutes before bedtime to relax and wind down. Read a good book, take a warm bath, or work on a hobby. That way you'll be calm, cool, and collected when you get into bed.

❖ **Don't push it.** You can't force yourself to sleep. If you've been lying in bed staring at the ceiling for more than a half hour, get up. Try to do some quiet activities, and then go back to bed. Repeat this as often as needed.

❖ **Warm milk may work.** Warm milk has been a home remedy for insomnia for years. Milk contains tryptophan, an amino acid that researchers say can help you sleep. Other foods high in tryptophan include meats, poultry, and beans.

The long-range plan for insomnia

Do you find yourself nodding off at awkward or even dangerous times during the day? If so, you need a long-range plan to make sure you get your sleep at night — not while on the job or at the wheel.

❖ **Comfort is the key.** In the fairy tale The Princess and the Pea, the princess couldn't sleep because she felt a pea underneath a hundred mattresses. While most people aren't quite that sensitive, it is much easier to snooze in a comfortable atmosphere. Make sure you have a good mattress, and wear comfortable clothes to bed. The temperature shouldn't be too hot or cold, and your bedroom should be quiet and dark to help you sleep.

❖ **Get in a rut.** While it may sound boring, getting into a sleep schedule "rut" can help you sleep better. Go to bed at the same time every night, and get up at the same time every morning.

❖ **Limit your in-bed activities.** If you use your bed to eat, read, watch television, or work, you may be asking for trouble. Going to bed should signal your body that it is time to go to sleep. If you use your bed for too many other activities, your body may get confused at bedtime. It won't automatically relax for sleep like it should.

❖ **Exercise for sound sleep.** Regular exercise can improve your snooze time. About 20 to 30 minutes of exercise three or four days a week should help, but avoid exercising just before bedtime.

❖ **Avoid alcohol, caffeine, and smoking.** You probably know that you shouldn't drink coffee before going to bed. Caffeine is a stimulant and can keep you awake. You may not realize that nicotine in cigarettes is also a stimulant. And although drinking alcohol may make you sleepy, it may also cause you to wake up during the night.

Jaw pain

Soreness in the muscles attaching the U-shaped bone of the lower face to the skull

Your jaw is one joint you probably take for granted but use millions of times each day. Moving your jaw is like walking or breathing — you don't think about it until it hurts. Like most of your other joints, the muscles connecting it will suffer the usual number of spasms and pains. But sometimes jaw pain is a signal of something more serious — injury, infection, a nerve disorder, or pain referred from somewhere else in your body.

 It's time to see your doctor if you have jaw pain and:

Pain when biting or chewing
Stiffness in your jaw
Loosened or damaged teeth
Numbness in your lower lip
Recent blow to the face

You will probably know if you have fractured your jaw. Because of the jaw's shape, a knock to your face or head can crack the bone on one side and cause injury to the other side as well. Get medical attention. You may need to have an X-ray.

- **Pain in front of your ear on one or both sides**
- **Your jaw extends further forward than normal**
- **Your mouth does not close properly**
- **Difficulty speaking**

These symptoms could mean you have dislocated your jaw. Usually this happens after a blow to the face, but it could result from something as simple as yawning. It is fairly easy to put the joint back into place, but you should still see your doctor since it is quite common for the dislocation to reoccur.

- **Swollen and painful gums**
- **Swollen lymph nodes in your neck**
- **Difficulty opening your mouth**

Usually, wisdom teeth, the four back molars, develop and erupt between the ages of 17 and 21, but sometimes they never fully emerge until later in life. If, as an older adult, you experience these symptoms, you may have a late-developing or impacted wisdom tooth. See your dentist.

- **Stuffy nose with a green-yellow discharge**
- **Tension, fullness, or pressure in your face and head**
- **Throbbing headache made worse by bending over**
- **Pain behind your eyes**
- **Pain behind your cheeks that feels like a toothache**
- **Loss of the sense of smell**
- **Fever and chills**
- **Cough or sore throat**

Your sinuses are air-filled pockets and passageways in the bones around your nose that connect your nose, eyes, and ears. When your sinuses become irritated and inflamed by allergies, pollution, smoke, or a viral infection, you can develop sinusitis. (See also *Nose, runny or stuffy* chapter.)

- Ache or throbbing pain in a tooth
- Pain when chewing or biting
- Swollen, red, and sore gum around tooth
- Swollen and tender glands in your neck and side of face
- Earache
- Fever
- Headache
- Bad-tasting discharge in your mouth

Bacteria sometime reach the nerves and blood vessels inside a tooth, or the area between the teeth and gums, causing an infection. If this infection spreads into the tissue and bone surrounding the tooth, it is called an abscess. See your dentist as soon as possible.

- Pressure-like pain in the center of your chest that can vary from mild to severe
- Pain in your throat, neck, gums, upper body, or left arm
- Discomfort in your chest and throat similar to indigestion
- Nausea
- Sweating
- Dizziness
- Difficulty breathing

These symptoms could mean you are suffering from angina pectoris. An angina attack occurs when the heart does not receive enough oxygen. This usually happens when the blood to the heart is insufficient due to coronary heart disease. This is not a heart attack. The pain is not as intense or lengthy as during a heart attack, and no heart muscle is damaged. You should consider the pain a warning sign and see your doctor immediately — you are at risk of a heart attack. (See also *Chest pain* chapter.)

- Muscles in your face and jaw that feel stiff or sore, especially in the morning
- Loose and sore teeth
- Headaches
- Muscle pain in your neck and shoulders
- Teeth that are extra sensitive to heat and cold
- A habit of clenching your teeth when under stress
- Inability to open your jaw completely

Bruxism is the medical term for tooth grinding. If you have the above symptoms, you may be spending your nights clenching, gritting, or grinding your teeth. Usually caused by stress, bruxism is an unconscious habit that can damage your teeth, gums, and jaw muscles. Your dentist can fit you with a biteplate that you wear at night. This won't keep you from grinding your teeth, but it will prevent most of the tooth damage that bruxism can cause. There are other steps you can take to rid yourself of this destructive habit. Ask your dentist for advice.

- Headache or an ache in the muscles in front of your ears
- Jaw joint sometimes gets stuck
- Clicking, cracking, or crunching noises when moving your jaw
- Pain when yawning
- Difficulty opening your mouth completely or moving your jaw from side to side
- Sore and swollen muscles around your jaw
- Hearing loss or a ringing, roaring, or buzzing sound in your ears

If you suffer from a mix of these symptoms, chances are you have been diagnosed with anything from a toothache to a migraine to a sinus infection. Many people come to believe they are suffering from a psychological problem since abnormalities don't always show up on lab tests or X-rays. But, like 20 million other Americans, you may have a very real condition called temporomandibular joint syndrome or TMJ.

Immediate help for temporomandibular joint syndrome (TMJ)

TMJ is a disorder that affects the joint connecting your lower jaw to your head. This "hinge" is very complicated and quite unstable, even though the muscles that work the jaw are among the most powerful in the body. When you think of the tremendous pressure you use when biting and chewing, and the range of motion that your jaw is capable of, it is no surprise that the joint is easily damaged.

The causes of TMJ are varied, and it can be difficult to diagnose. They include:

❖ A blow to your head or face, causing a partial dislocation of the jaw

❖ Whiplash

❖ Clenching or grinding teeth caused by tension

❖ Misaligned teeth that cause the jaw to shift in order to line up the bite

❖ Poorly fitting dentures

❖ Poor posture

❖ Arthritis

❖ The habit of cradling a phone receiver between your ear and neck

A big step in successful treatment of TMJ is an accurate diagnosis. Once you have identified the source of your pain, you can move on to relieving it.

❖ **Unclench.** Clenching your jaw is a habit. You may do it a thousand times a day and not even be aware of it. Everyone reacts to the stresses of life differently, but if you find that you clench your jaw when you are tense, angry, or upset, try channeling that energy into something not so destructive, like squeezing a soft rubber ball or whistling.

❖ **Stop grinding your teeth.** This is another habit you may not even know you have, but if your spouse says you grind your teeth in your sleep, see your dentist. She can fit you with a nighttime mouthpiece that will force your jaws apart.

- ❖ **Ice it down** — heat it up. Cold compresses followed by moist heat can ease the spasms in your jaw muscles.

- ❖ **Rub it out.** Massaging the muscles in your neck, back, shoulders, and face can soothe the soreness and relax the tension.

- ❖ **Easy does it.** After you've warmed up your face with compresses and massage, stretch your jaw muscles, but do it gently. You want to relieve the muscle spasms that accompany TMJ, not cause further injury.

- ❖ **Toss that pillow and turn over.** The way you sleep at night can affect how you feel the next day. Using pillows and sleeping on your stomach puts an unnatural strain on your neck. Instead, roll up a soft towel, place it under your neck, and then sleep on your back.

- ❖ **Pull your triggers.** Certain activities will trigger muscle spasms in your jaw, causing the joint to lock up. Try to avoid whatever causes you pain. For instance, if you feel a yawn coming on, place your fist under your chin to keep your mouth from opening too wide.

- ❖ **Get rid of the gum.** Chewing gum will only irritate already sore, overused muscles.

- ❖ **Bag the bagels.** Hard, chewy foods will make your jaw work harder. Try softening up your diet.

- ❖ **Stop the swelling.** Over-the-counter pain relievers, like ibuprofen, will not only make you more comfortable, they will ease the inflammation in your damaged jaw muscles.

- ❖ **Listen to your body.** Certain foods and drugs can increase the tension in some people by speeding up their metabolisms. Caffeine and decongestants are two examples. If coffee tends to make you a little jittery, you could end up unconsciously clenching your jaw even more, so cut back or switch to decaf. If your cold medicine is making you jumpy, try another product. Your jaw will thank you.

The long-range plan for temporomandibular joint syndrome (TMJ)

The preceding suggestions are relatively easy changes to make in your lifestyle, a small price to pay for less pain. But if you are still suffering from the effects of TMJ, even after trying these conservative approaches, you may need more radical treatment.

❖ **Dial your dentist.** If the shape of your jaw or the alignment of your teeth is the cause of your TMJ, you may have no choice but to seek professional help. Your dentist can fit you with a custom mouthguard that will take the pressure off your jaw muscles and allow the spasms to relax, or he might recommend orthodontics to move your teeth into their proper position. He can also grind the surfaces of your teeth to allow them to match up more evenly. If all else fails, he might recommend orthopedic surgery to shift your jaw bone. Don't rush into these last procedures. Think over all your options and get a second opinion.

❖ **Learn to cope.** Counseling and special training may be necessary to teach you how to relax and to provide you with more effective ways of handling stress.

Joint pain

Discomfort or achiness in your ankles, knees, hips, shoulders, fingers, wrists, elbows, or neck

Every move we make depends on some joint performing properly, whether it's lifting groceries from the car or doing a back-bending dip dancing the tango. But, like breathing, we take this function of our bodies for granted, usually until something goes wrong. You are lucky, indeed, if you haven't experienced joint pain sometime in your life. Usually a hot bath, an aspirin, and a good night's sleep can set things right. If not, you may need an expert diagnosis.

It's time to see your doctor if you have joint pain and:

- Recent injury
- Swelling
- Restricted movement of a joint

If you have damaged the ligaments holding the bones together, you may have dislocated a joint. Your doctor may have to manipulate the joint in order to line the bones up correctly. Surgery might be necessary if you repeatedly dislocate it.

- Fever and chills

You may have an infection that needs immediate medical care. Lyme disease is one example of a bacterial infection that affects the joints.

- Inflammation of a joint
- Limited movement of the joint
- Injury or strain to the joint within a week of symptoms

Bursae are small, fluid-filled sacs that act as cushions between the working parts of your joints. When you injure or strain a joint, these bursae can become inflamed. This is called bursitis. (See also *Hip pain* chapter.)

- Swelling
- Warmth in affected area
- Muscle pain or tenderness that increases with motion

If you have these symptoms you may have tendinitis, an inflammation of one of your tendons. It is often caused by an injury, or by repeating the same motion over and over. (See also *Arm, elbow, or shoulder pain* chapter.)

- Redness and swelling in your joint
- Severe pain that usually occurs at night

Gout is a form of acute arthritis marked by inflammation of the joints. It is caused by too much uric acid in the blood, which forms crystals in the joints. Attacks usually last about a week.

- Morning joint stiffness
- Limited movement and dexterity

This could mean osteoarthritis, a condition where the cartilage in your joints gradually breaks down. Usually, you will feel an aching pain when you move or put weight on your joints. (See also **Knee pain** chapter.)

- Swelling and redness in your joint
- Low fever
- General ill-feeling
- Severe morning stiffness that can last for hours

These symptoms may indicate the onset of rheumatoid arthritis, a disease that inflames the joints. Resting may not bring you relief from the pain.

Immediate help for arthritis

Approximately 37 million Americans suffer from arthritis, which means "inflammation of the joint." It can be caused by more than 100 different diseases, and, in most cases, has no cure. Even though doctors routinely prescribe antibiotics, anti-inflammatories, and other types of drugs, the best treatment may come from you. By adjusting your lifestyle and taking responsibility for managing your pain, you can lead a normal, productive life.

The first step in treating your arthritis is to make sure your problem is diagnosed correctly. Since many conditions have joint pain as a symptom, it is important to first rule out any serious illness, such as Lyme disease,

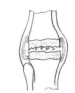

Normal Knee
Joint

Osteoarthritic

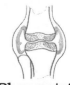

Rheumatoid

scleroderma, lupus, and others. Once you know you are dealing with arthritis, you can begin treatment.

- ❖ **Become arthritis smart.** Studies show that arthritis sufferers who learn about the disease have a better outlook on their future, and are better able to adjust their lifestyles and manage the pain. So go to the library and read as many books and journals as you can find. Join the Arthritis Foundation, find a support group through your doctor or hospital, or contact your local college or university. Understanding arthritis gives you better weapons for the battle.

- ❖ **A little rest goes a long way.** Acute attacks of arthritis pain require rest. The joints need to settle from the swelling, and you can take the time to pamper your body with a heating pad or ice pack. But don't get too comfortable. It's important to get out of bed and on with your life.

- ❖ **Perfect your posture.** While standing or sitting, adjust your body so your back is straight, your neck is at a natural angle, and your feet rest comfortably on the floor. If you put your joints in stressful positions, you'll just strain them and aggravate your arthritis.

- ❖ **Do some shift work.** Whether typing, sewing, writing a letter, or balancing the checkbook, don't let a few moments turn into an hour. If you stay in one position too long, your joints can stiffen up and start to hurt. So get up, walk around, and stretch your muscles once in a while.

- ❖ **Spare your joints.** During your day, think about how you use your joints to perform each task. Instead of gripping or twisting with your fingers, hold things with your palms. Take advantage of modern appliances such as electric can openers and knives. Let your stronger joints and muscles carry your burdens. For instance, use a fanny pack instead of a shoulder purse; lead with your stronger leg when climbing stairs. Take a careful look around your home or workplace. If necessary, rearrange shelves, tools, equipment, and appliances to reduce bending, lifting and carrying.

❖ **Take two.** Aspirin or ibuprofen will help relieve your pain and reduce swelling in your joints.

❖ **Investigate supplements.** Experts constantly test various supplements on conditions like arthritis. While not all the results are conclusive, many recommendations are worth a try. For instance, osteoarthritis sufferers can take folic acid with vitamin B12 to help give them a stronger grip. And if you have rheumatoid arthritis, you might try eating more fish, like lake trout, mackerel, and herring. It will give your body some much-needed omega-3 fatty acids to help you fight this crippling disease.

The long-range plan for arthritis

Chronic arthritis may mean facing the condition every day for the rest of your life. Whether or not you control the disease depends on how you approach it.

❖ **Lose weight.** Extra pounds mean extra pressure on your joints, which can lead to more pain. Work with your doctor on a safe weight-loss program.

❖ **Exercise wisely.** Experts agree that a regular, gentle exercise program will improve your overall health and fitness without harming your joints. It will give you stronger bones and muscles, more flexible joints, more energy, better sleep, weight control, improved sense of well-being, and a greater feeling of hope and optimism. Your doctor, physical therapist, or occupational therapist can show you specific exercises for your condition, but in general, you should include flexibility, strengthening, and endurance exercises.

Flexibility, or range of motion, exercises are gentle stretches and movements that keep your joints supple so you can stay up with your day-to-day activities. But don't think you can substitute your daily chores for a regular exercise program. Sweeping the floor or making the beds will not work your joints fully.

Strengthening exercises will improve your muscle tone and help keep your joints stable. The two most common types are easy to do practically anywhere. With isometric exercises, you repeatedly tense and relax certain sets of muscles, without moving any part of your body. Isotonic exercises require you to flex a muscle by moving a joint, for example lifting your foot while sitting in a chair. Your doctor can advise you on speed, weight, and number of repetitions.

Endurance exercises will benefit your entire body, including your heart and lungs. You should start slow and easy with these, but you can build up to 30 minutes per day, three times a week. Examples of good endurance exercises are walking, swimming or water aerobics, and bicycling.

Some tips for making your exercise plan more enjoyable are:

- Find the time of day that suits you best. If a routine bores you, vary the schedule.
- Warm up by massaging your muscles or applying heat to sore joints, then begin with your flexibility exercises.
- Dress in loose comfortable clothes and well-supported shoes.
- Keep to a steady pace, one that doesn't place too much stress on your body.
- Breathe. Try counting out loud to help you take deep breaths.
- Don't push yourself. You don't want to be in pain the following day, so start out easy and gradually increase your endurance. Stop if you feel pain, dizziness, or nausea.
- Set goals you can meet, and record your progress.
- Don't skip a day, even if your arthritis flares up. Just cut back on some of the more strenuous exercises.
- Accept no excuses. Make exercise a part of your life, and it will stop feeling like work.

You can ease your arthritis pain by seeking out even more ways to adapt to your condition. Explore pain management programs that teach relaxation, meditation, and guided imagery. Look for labor-saving products and devices developed with people just like you in mind. Examine everything around you; you'll be surprised how small changes can improve the quality of your life.

Arthritis exercises

Check with your doctor or physical therapist before starting any exercise program.

❖ **Arm Raises.** While standing or lying on your back, slowly swing your arm straight out in front of you and up over your head. Reach for the sky for a moment, then slowly lower your arm back down to your side. Repeat with your other arm.

❖ **Shoulder Stretch.** Sit or stand tall. Reach one hand behind your head and down to the middle of your back. Your elbow should be pointing to the ceiling. Reach your other hand behind your waist and up to the middle of your back. That elbow should be pointing to the floor. Gently stretch, trying to join your hands. Switch arm positions and repeat.

❖ **Ankle Flex.** Sit with your feet comfortably placed on the floor. Alternate lifting your toes then your heels as high as possible. Make sure you feel the stretch in your ankle.

❖ **Finger Curls.** Stretch your fingers wide apart, then curl just your fingertips down so they touch the top of your palm. Stretch your thumb by touching it to your little finger. Open your hand and repeat.

❖ **Neck Stretch.** Keeping your head straight, pull your chin back into your neck. Hold that position for a few seconds, then, without raising your shoulders, stretch your neck by lifting the top of your head toward the ceiling.

❖ **Praying Hands.** Place your palms together and bring them into your chest so that your fingers are pointing toward the ceiling and your elbows are straight out to the side. Try to bend your wrists into a ninety degree angle. Gently push your palms against each other without moving either hand. Count to five slowly then relax.

❖ **Knee Pull.** Lie on your back. Stretch one leg out straight on the floor and bend the knee of the other. Now grasp the thigh of your straight leg and pull that knee into your chest. Straighten the leg, pointing your heel toward the ceiling, then lower it to the floor. Repeat with your other leg. Don't force the movements if you feel pain.

❖ **Leg Roll.** Lie on your back. Keeping your leg straight and your foot flexed, roll your leg out so that your toes are pointing to the side. Gently push the side of your foot to the floor. You should feel a stretch in your calf and your hip. Roll the leg back and, for an isometric exercise, push the back of your knee down into the floor. Hold this for a few seconds then relax. Repeat with your other leg.

Knee pain

Dull ache in the knee
Sharp pain with movement of the knee joint

Swivel, bend, slide, glide. If you were keeping track of your knee movements all day, this is probably the pattern you would find. Your knee joint is the largest joint in your body and probably the most complex. With all our modern technology, no machine can come close to doing all the amazing things it does. Unfortunately, just like a machine, your knees can gradually break down after years of use. They also can be easily injured. The result — pain, swelling, stiffness, and an end to many of your favorite activities.

 ## It's time to see your doctor if you have knee pain and:

- You've injured your knee within the past 24 hours
- Your knee is misshapen
- You're unable to move or put weight on it

It's possible you have a fracture, dislocation, or serious injury. Get medical treatment at once.

- Redness, tenderness, and swelling
- Pain that usually occurs at night and becomes so severe you can't get relief

These are the symptoms of gout, a form of acute arthritis marked by inflammation of the joints. It usually begins in the knee or foot and is caused by too much uric acid in the blood, which forms crystals in the joints. Attacks usually last about a week.

- Tenderness and limited movement
- Worse pain when knee is bent

246

Fever (sometimes)

This could indicate bursitis, an inflammation of the soft tissue around your knee joint. Rest, along with aspirin or aspirin substitute, should clear up the problem in a few weeks. If the pain persists, see your doctor. (See also *Hip pain* chapter.)

Fever and chills

You may have an infection that needs immediate medical care. Lyme disease is one example of a bacterial infection that inflames the joints, often the knee.

A locked-up joint

Sometimes, even minor twisting can tear your cartilage and cause pain. Athletes often suffer this type of injury. If your knee locks up so you can't fully straighten or bend it, or "gives way," you need to see your doctor.

Morning joint stiffness
Limited movement and dexterity

This could mean osteoarthritis, a condition where the cartilage in your joints gradually breaks down. Usually, you will feel an aching pain when you move or put weight on your joints.

Immediate help for osteoarthritis

Living with this painful condition can be a challenge. Since so much of your daily life involves moving around, it can be frustrating to feel limited by the pain of arthritis. What can you do for some quick relief?

❖ **Lift that leg.** Elevate your knee above heart level to help reduce painful swelling.

❖ **Soothe your soreness.** A warm heating pad will help relieve your aching knee. Apply it to your joints for 20 minutes two to three times a day. Haven't got one? Try filling a clean, dry, cotton sock with uncooked rice and tieing the end closed. Heat it in your microwave for three minutes, and you now have a flexible heating pad that will conform to any aching part of your body. The sock will stay warm for up to an hour, and you don't have to worry about burns.

❖ **Tape your kneecap.** Taping your kneecap to the inside of your leg may sound strange, but it actually helps relieve pressure caused by a misaligned knee. It's also a safe, inexpensive way to make climbing stairs and walking a little easier. After pulling your kneecap toward the inner part of your leg, tape it so the two end pieces of the tape are on the outer side of your leg, not touching each other. The best tape to use is a roll of 2-inch-wide athletic adhesive tape.

❖ **Consider a cane.** Using a cane in the hand opposite your painful knee will reduce the force on your joint by up to 50 percent. Try it for a few days to see if it helps.

The long-range plan for osteoarthritis

You can usually relieve the symptoms of osteoarthritis but, unfortunately, any deterioration in your joints will be permanent. By making some changes in your lifestyle, you can have more control over this painful condition.

❖ **Balance your diet.** It's important to eat well for general health, but certain foods also may have a special impact on osteoarthritis. A vegetarian diet may especially help, but simply eating more fruits and vegetables and less meat could help relieve your arthritis. The omega-3 fatty acids in deep-water fish, such as salmon, mackerel, tuna, and herring, are also known to relieve arthritis. You may want to try eliminating dairy products from your diet to see if your symptoms improve. Some researchers think dairy products and other foods, such as wheat and black walnuts, may trigger arthritis.

❖ **Exercise regularly.** It may be tough to work out when your joints are aching, but exercise helps your knees stay mobile and strengthens the muscles around them. Although doctors used to recommend rest for arthritis sufferers, they now think even aerobic exercise can be valuable. Exercises that aren't weight bearing, such as bicycling, swimming, and water aerobics, are good choices. If you prefer vigorous aerobic exercise, and your knees can tolerate it, go for it. You need to find your own best level of fitness, but be sure to check with your doctor and physical therapist before doing anything too strenuous. Besides giving you greater strength and physical well-being, exercise can give you a greater feeling of control over your arthritis.

❖ **Battle back with vitamins.** Vitamins C, E, and beta-carotene can go to bat for you in your battle against knee pain. Researchers have found these potent antioxidants may help keep the osteoarthritis in your knees from getting worse. Vitamin D may also help painful knees by strengthening the bones around them. This keeps you from getting bone-weakening cavities and cysts. Next time you go grocery shopping, be sure to fill your cart with plenty of fresh fruits, green and yellow vegetables, nuts, seeds, and wheat germ. And don't forget to enjoy plenty of sunshine.

Your knees are the key to such simple motions as standing up, walking, climbing, or kicking. Whether you're an active athlete or someone who simply likes to dance or ride a bike, you have the potential to develop knee problems. By keeping your leg muscles strong and taking care of your health, you should find your knees supporting you well into old age.

Leg pain

Aches or sharp pains in the muscles of the legs

Leg pain can range from occasional cramps to chronic muscle spasms. Everything from too much exercise to unhealthy clots restricting your blood flow can cause you to grit your teeth and grasp your leg in agony. If your legs cramp up at night or after a hard workout, try gentle stretches before bedtime and take some time to cool down after exercising.

If your legs feel like they're creeping, squirming, or aching every time they're still, you may have restless legs syndrome. These sensations stop when you move, so you may end up shaking your legs constantly, which can lead to another problem — insomnia. Restless legs syndrome may be caused by iron deficiency anemia, pregnancy, rheumatoid arthritis, and the use of antidepressants and other medicines. Although bothersome, it's generally harmless and may come and go over the years.

Serious leg problems could result from such conditions as blood clots, varicose veins, phlebitis, or intermittent claudication. These conditions, which are discussed in the following section, may require a doctor's care and a long-term investment in caring for your legs. Diabetes and cigarette smoking are two causes of such problems. Watch for other clues such as diagnosed atherosclerosis; high blood pressure; high cholesterol; and a family history of stroke, heart disease, or vascular disease.

It's time to see your doctor if you have leg pain and:

- Enlarged veins in your legs
- Pain, swelling, and a persistent itch in the affected area
- Thin, hard, dry, discolored skin

You might have a condition called varicose veins. This occurs when veins in your legs become swollen and twisted. They will appear larger and much bluer than normal. There are various causes of the condition but few treatments besides surgery.

- Pain and tenderness along a vein
- Skin discoloration and swelling
- Rapid pulse

- Low-grade fever
- Joint pain

These are symptoms of phlebitis, a vein inflammation that sometimes occurs in acute or chronic infections or following surgery or childbirth. It also may develop from varicose veins.

- Pain in the ankle, calf, or thigh that does not go away with rest
- Tenderness and redness in the leg/foot area
- Pain when walking, raising your leg, or flexing your foot
- Fever
- Rapid heartbeat

Sometimes after a long period of bed rest due to surgery or illness, blood pools in your veins, especially in the legs. In the case of deep-vein thrombosis, a clot forms within the veins of the lower legs and restricts blood flow. Being overweight, smoking, and taking estrogen increase your risk of deep-vein thrombosis.

- Tingling and numbness
- Weakened muscles
- Shooting pains at night
- Ulcers on your toes or fingers
- Pale, dry, and sensitive skin
- Weight loss

If these symptoms gradually appear over several months and spread throughout your body, you might have peripheral neuropathy, a disease of the nerves. This can result from a reaction to drugs or chemicals, or it could be a complication of another problem. It is important to identify the cause and correct it if possible. (See also *Foot pain* chapter.)

- Stomach pain
- Itchy skin
- Fatigue and paleness
- Muscle cramps
- "Fishy" breath

If you have these symptoms, along with numbness, burning, and tingling in your legs and feet, you may have chronic kidney failure.

- **Aches and cramping during exercise that stop when you rest**
- **Minor injuries that don't heal**
- **Chronic skin ulcerations**
- **Sudden onset of pain, coolness, and numbness in the affected limb**

This could be intermittent claudication, a condition where your heart is unable to pump enough blood to your legs. It's a symptom of serious artery disease.

Immediate help for leg pain

You can take care of minor leg pain and cramps by using common-sense remedies like rest, gentle stretching, and mild pain relievers as needed.

- ❖ **Lower your leg.** Help the blood circulate to your leg by keeping it lower than the rest of your body. If your pain is worse at night, you may get some relief by hanging your leg over the side of the bed.
- ❖ **Keep it warm.** Cover your leg with clothing or blankets, soak it in a hot bath, or use a heating pad, but don't overdo it. Excessive heat may enlarge your blood vessels too much, which can affect your deeper circulation.
- ❖ **Flex, don't rub.** When you get a cramp or "charley horse," your first impulse is to grab your leg and try to rub it out. Instead, sit down, straighten out your leg, grab the ball of your foot, and stretch it toward you. Hold that position until you feel the cramp relax. Be sure to stretch your calf muscles every day to help prevent charley horse spasms.
- ❖ **Consider quinine.** High doses of quinine seem to help nighttime leg cramps, but it also can cause serious side effects, such as ringing in the ears, deafness, mental confusion, disturbed vision, vertigo, headache, nausea, and vomiting. Consult with your doctor before taking quinine.

Help for varicose veins

Do your legs look like an overused road map? If so, you're probably suffering from varicose veins, an unsightly and often painful condition. Varicose veins are twisted, bulging blood vessels caused by blood backing up in a vein.

Varicose veins can be removed surgically, but the problem may return if you don't deal with the underlying causes. Here are some things you can do to prevent or relieve varicose veins:

❖ **Avoid long periods of standing.** Standing increases the pressure in your veins. If you're overweight, try to shed those excess pounds. Obesity increases pressure that can block blood flow in the veins or decrease support for the veins themselves.

❖ **Elevate your legs.** Resting with your feet raised higher than your hips helps your blood circulate back to your heart. When you sit, don't cross your legs because this cuts off your circulation.

❖ **Exercise.** Walking improves leg and vein strength, but any exercise that keeps your muscles pumping is good. Heavy aerobic exercise may cause discomfort.

❖ **Elasticize.** Support hosiery can provide immediate relief from the itching and aching often associated with varicose veins. They're made so most of the pressure is on your ankle, with less at midcalf and midthigh. This helps keep the blood flowing back to your heart. If your problem is severe, your doctor may prescribe custom-made compression stockings. Both types of stockings should be put on first thing in the morning before blood pools in your feet and ankles.

The long-range plan for leg pain

Serious conditions like intermittent claudication can have grave consequences if allowed to go untreated.

Claudication's main symptom is pain in your calf or thigh muscle when you walk, which stops when you rest. It usually results from narrow arteries that restrict the supply of blood to your muscles. When you're resting, enough blood flows to the muscle to meet its needs, so the pain subsides. As this disease gets worse, you may have trouble keeping your foot warm, and you may only be able to relieve the pain by dangling your leg or not using it at all. Minor cuts, burns, and injuries on your foot and leg will heal slowly, and you may develop skin ulcers. Attacking this problem involves exercising and adopting a healthy lifestyle.

❖ **Pound the pavement.** If someone told you to walk until you couldn't stand the pain, you'd probably think he was crazy. But, believe it or not, exercise is the best way to relieve the pain of intermittent claudication. Walk until it hurts, then rest for several minutes until the pain subsides. Walk again, then rest, and keep alternating for about an hour. By walking one hour three times a week, you should experience less pain within two or three months.

❖ **Check your AAA.** No, not your automobile club. AAA stands for abdominal aortic aneurysm, a weakness in the wall of the artery that supplies blood to your stomach, liver, spleen, and legs. If your artery ruptures, your chances of survival are low. Intermittent claudication is a common sign of this condition, which affects almost one out of every 10 men over age 65. All men in this age group should be screened for this condition every year. Start earlier if you get severe pain in your calf muscles when you walk.

❖ **Stop smoking.** Studies show that smokers who quit have less leg pain when exercising and at rest.

❖ **Watch your diet.** Keep your cholesterol level down. This condition often results from clogged arteries caused by a build-up of cholesterol and other fatty materials. Other risk factors include diabetes and high blood pressure.

Menstrual changes

Spotting between periods
Heavy bleeding during periods
Missing periods

Although being a woman has its good points, it has certain drawbacks as well. Most women consider their monthly period to be one of those drawbacks. If you're lucky enough to escape the pain, bloating, and irritability that many women experience, your menstrual period can still be messy, inconvenient, and annoying.

However, it is a natural occurrence, and if something about your menstrual period changes, you need to take note. If you are of child-bearing age, and the normal time for your period comes and goes without a spot, you're probably pregnant. If you are older, you may be entering menopause.

On the other hand, if you bleed between periods, you may be reacting to a prescription drug such as birth control pills, or you could have something more serious, like cancer of the reproductive system.

It's time to see the doctor if you have:

- Tenderness or swelling in your lower abdomen, possibly accompanied by a hard mass that can be felt through your skin
- Upset stomach
- Symptoms of anemia (fatigue, paleness, shortness of breath)
- Unexplained weight loss
- Deepening of your voice and excessive growth of body hair
- Painful intercourse

This combination of symptoms could indicate ovarian cancer.

⠿ **Spotting between periods or after sex**
You may have cervical polyps, which usually cause no pain, but may need to be removed surgically.

⠿ **Sweating, hot flashes**
⠿ **Vaginal dryness**
⠿ **Irregular periods**
⠿ **Breast pain**
⠿ **Depression, insomnia, nervousness**
If you're the right age, these symptoms could mean you are entering menopause.

Immediate help for menopause

You dealt with it all of your adult life, and you thought you'd be so relieved when you didn't have to worry about having a menstrual period ever again. It was one of the few things about getting older that actually seemed appealing. However, now that you've stopped having periods, you've discovered that menopause comes with its own unique set of problems. You're as irritable and depressed as you ever were before your period, you break into an embarrassing sweat for no apparent reason, and sex has become difficult and sometimes even painful because your vagina is so dry. Fortunately, menopause is a temporary condition, and you can defend yourself from some of its side effects.

Your menopausal symptoms are caused by hormonal changes. During your 40s, your ovaries gradually produce less estrogen, and your periods may become irregular. Your periods will stop completely around the age of 52, and you will officially enter menopause. After you have gone a year without a period, you are considered postmenopausal.

The years leading up to postmenopause can be difficult, and many women choose hormone replacement therapy (HRT) to help ease the transition from their childbearing years to their golden years. Hormone replacement therapy can do more than just cool down your hot flashes. When your body slows its production of estrogen, it puts you more at risk for heart disease. But replacing your estrogen through HRT can cut your risk of heart disease in half.

Estrogen also works to keep your bones strong. So when your estrogen levels drop during menopause, you may lose bone density and increase your risk of osteoporosis. HRT can help protect you against the bone-shattering effects of this disease. Unfortunately, HRT seems to put you more at risk for breast cancer, and it slightly increases your risk of blood clots.

You have to weigh the benefits against the risks when deciding whether you want to try HRT. If you are at a high risk for heart disease or osteoporosis, HRT may be just what you need. On the other hand, if you've had breast cancer or are at high risk for the disease, you may want to find alternatives to HRT. You're considered

Benefits of HRT

❖ Eases menopause symptoms like hot flashes and vaginal dryness

❖ Cuts your risk of heart disease in half

❖ Lowers your risk of osteoporosis

❖ Helps keep your skin from sagging and wrinkling

❖ Helps prevent excessive hair growth

Risks associated with HRT

❖ Increases your risk of breast cancer

❖ Slightly increases your risk of blood clots

❖ Estrogen alone can increase your risk of endometrial (lining of your uterus) cancer

❖ May cause side effects like breast swelling or tenderness, water retention, or unusual bleeding

❖ Not recommended for women with liver disease

high risk if you've had a relative with breast cancer, began your menstrual period at an early age, had no children, or went through menopause late in life.

If you developed blood clots while you were pregnant or taking birth control pills, HRT also may not be a good choice for you. Discuss the possibilities thoroughly with your doctor before making your decision.

The long-range plan for menopause

You want relief from your hot flashes and other menopausal symptoms, but you've considered it carefully, and decided you don't want hormone replacement therapy. Perhaps your doctor advised against it because you've had breast cancer, or perhaps you just don't like the idea of taking medicine every day, and you want a more natural alternative. The answer to your dilemma may come from the East.

Women in Far East countries like China and Japan experience menopause symptoms far less than women in other parts of the world. Research shows that the high amount of soy in the Asian diet may be responsible for this lack of hot flashes and depression during menopause. People in those countries eat about 20 to 50 times more soy than people in the United States.

Soy contains *phytoestrogens*, plant estrogens which may act like a weak form of human estrogen when you eat it. Many other plants contain phytoestrogens, but soy has a particularly strong type called isoflavones. Because these isoflavones can act like estrogen in your body, they may help perform the same duties as HRT, only without the risks and side effects. In fact, while HRT increases your risk of breast cancer, soy may actually lower your risk of that disease. Among soy's many health benefits:

❖ **Lowers cholesterol levels.** Studies show that eating six servings of soy foods a week can reduce your cholesterol by 20 percent. This reduction in cholesterol can lead to healthier arteries and a healthier heart.

❖ **Fends off osteoporosis.** One of the biggest concerns women have when going through menopause is the effect of osteoporosis on their bones. The best way to fight that is to get plenty of calcium. Tofu and yogurt are the two best sources of bone-guarding calcium recommended by the Osteoporosis Foundation.

❖ **Cuts down cancer.** Breast cancer isn't the only type of cancer that soy can help you avoid. Research indicates that soy may provide protection against other cancers as well, particularly cancer of the prostate and colon.

❖ **Provides protein.** Everyone needs protein, but when you get most of your protein from animal sources like beef, you're getting lots of fat as well. While soy also has some fat, it contains polyunsaturated fat, which is much better for you than the saturated fat you'll get from a hamburger.

If you want natural relief from menopausal symptoms, try some tofu, soy milk, soy cheese, soy sauce, or textured vegetable protein made from soy. The taste may surprise and delight you, and you'll be getting lots of disease-fighting power as well.

Mouth dryness

Excessive thirst
Lack of saliva
Difficulty talking or swallowing

Everyone who is afraid of making speeches (and that's most people, according to recent polls) has experienced the dry mouth of nervousness. It's nothing to worry about — it's just a normal symptom of anxiety. Having a drier mouth is also a normal part of aging. Dry mouth can be a side effect of many prescription and non-prescription drugs, and the result of eating lots of salty food. But sometimes a dry mouth can signal that something more serious is going on in your body, and you need your doctor's help.

It's time to see your doctor if you have mouth dryness and:

- Excessive thirst
- Weak, rapid pulse
- Cool, sweaty skin
- Dizziness
- Muscle cramps or weakness
- Nausea or vomiting

You may have heat exhaustion, which means you've failed to drink enough to replace body fluids and salt you've lost through sweating. Drink liquids and seek medical care immediately.

- Severe thirst
- Dry lips
- Little or no urine
- Sunken eyes
- Muscle cramps or weakness
- Lightheadedness
- Rapid heart rate and breathing

These symptoms are a sign of dehydration, a common condition in older people. It can lead to more serious, sometimes fatal, conditions such as heat exhaustion and heatstroke.

- Excessive thirst
- Increased appetite
- Frequent urination
- Unexplained weight loss
- Frequent infections
- Fatigue

These symptoms may mean that you have diabetes.

- Fever
- Swollen and painful lymph glands on your neck
- Swelling and pain under your tongue or behind your ears
- Pus draining into your mouth

These are the signs of an infected salivary gland. A chronic illness or vitamin deficiency due to a poor diet can make you vulnerable to the bacteria that cause infections such as this one. Your doctor may prescribe an antibiotic to fight the infection.

- Constant dryness of your nose and eyes
- Vaginal dryness that makes intercourse painful
- Painful, achy joints

These symptoms may point to Sjogren's syndrome, an autoimmune disorder.

Immediate help for Sjogren's syndrome

Sjogren's syndrome affects between 200,000 and 4 million people in the United States. Most of the people affected are over the age of 50, and 90 percent are women. Named for the Swedish doctor who identified it in 1933, Sjogren's syndrome is an autoimmune disorder, which means that it causes your body to work against itself. Sjogren's destroys the glands that secrete mucous in your body, including the ones that produce tears in your eyes and saliva in your mouth. Although this is not a life-threatening disease, it does get progressively worse, and it can damage your eyes and mouth if the symptoms aren't treated.

Sjogren's syndrome can be either primary or secondary. Primary means it is a condition by itself, and it affects mostly your eyes and mouth. Secondary means it's a side effect of another autoimmune disease such as rheumatoid arthritis or lupus.

Sometimes it's difficult to diagnose Sjogren's syndrome because the symptoms may be vague at first and don't always happen at the same time. Along with the symptoms above, people with Sjogren's may experience burning tongue and throat, gritty eyes, tooth decay, digestive problems, dry skin, lung problems, kidney problems, muscular weakness, and extreme fatigue.

No one knows what causes Sjogren's syndrome. It may be related to heredity, hormones, or a virus that lies quietly in your body until it is suddenly triggered. If your doctor diagnoses your symptoms as Sjogren's syndrome, there are things you can do to make your life easier and keep yourself more comfortable.

* **Moisten your mouth with milk.** A recent study showed that drinking small sips of milk throughout the day, as well as drinking milk at meals, helped people with Sjogren's feel more comfortable. It also helped prevent tooth decay.

* **Chew on this.** Gum that contains the sugar substitute xylitol can be found at any supermarket checkout counter. Xylitol stimulates your saliva naturally, so it's an easy, inexpensive, and tasty way to help your dry mouth.

* **Try a tablet.** If your Sjogren's syndrome is not severe, over-the-counter tablets may help stimulate your own saliva. These orange-flavored tablets contain the sweetener sorbitol, along with calcium phosphate to protect the minerals in your teeth.

* **Send in a substitute.** You also can take advantage of several products designed to substitute for your own saliva. They are the most effective way to moisten a severely parched throat and mouth. Some even contain fluoride to protect your teeth from decay. Look for those with the American Dental Association seal of approval.

The long-range plan for Sjogren's syndrome

* **Get good professional care.** Be sure to see your doctor and dentist regularly so you can stay ahead of any problems that Sjogren's syndrome might cause. Tooth decay is a particular concern because you have no saliva to protect your teeth. So it's important to keep your mouth and teeth as clean and well-cared-for as possible.

* **Drink more liquids.** This is especially important at mealtime, when your saliva may not be enough to moisten your food.

* **Avoid drugs that dry.** Anticholinergics, antihistamines, and decongestants are among the drugs that will dry out your mucous membranes. Stay away from these drugs, or ask your doctor or pharmacist for a substitute. Also ask your doctor if dryness is a side effect of any new drug she prescribes for you.

❖ **Use a humidifier.** Moist air will be kinder to your dry mouth and eyes. Try to avoid air conditioning as well. It dries out the air and can irritate tender mucous membranes.

❖ **Watch your diet.** Don't let the discomfort of Sjogren's syndrome cause you to miss out on good nutrition. If your mouth is too sore at times to eat properly, try a liquid protein substitute, available at grocery and discount stores. You must eat well to keep up your strength and health.

Whether your dry mouth is a result of chronic illness or just a temporary challenge, it's an aggravating aspect of life. But today, more than ever before, you have a variety of ways to wet your whistle. Try our tips above and accept your dry mouth with a sense of humor, and you'll soon be whistling a happier tune.

Mouth or tongue soreness

Ulcers on your lips, tongue, or inside of your mouth
Pain, redness, or inflammation of your tongue

Nothing is as irritating as a sore in your mouth. It can interfere with talking, eating, even a romantic kiss. If you find yourself with this problem, first examine your oral hygiene habits. Are you brushing and flossing properly? Perhaps all you need is a softer toothbrush or a more regular routine. Then do a quick examination in the mirror. Are any of your teeth rubbing against your tongue or cheek? Has a filling or piece of tooth chipped off, leaving a ragged edge? Your dentist can fix these problems in a flash. If, however, you can't see any reason for a lingering soreness, you need an expert diagnosis.

It's time to see your doctor if you have mouth or tongue soreness and:

- A single small, pale lump on your tongue or mouth
- Any ulcer in your mouth that lasts longer than two weeks
- Any swelling in the mouth, tongue, or gum area
- Stiffness or loss of control of your tongue

This could indicate a tumor. Have your doctor perform a biopsy to determine if it is benign or malignant.

- White, sometimes swollen patches on the tongue or mouth
- Burning feeling in your mouth and throat
- Fever and chills

These symptoms signal candidiasis, a type of fungal infection that can affect your skin, nails, or any area with mucous membranes. If you have difficulty swallowing, the infection may have moved down into your esophagus.

- Pale, smooth tongue with redness on the tip and sides
- Fatigue
- Headaches
- Weak nails
- Breathlessness

These symptoms could indicate you have iron-deficiency anemia, the most common form of anemia. You could be losing too much iron from your system due to abnormally heavy bleeding, or your body may not be absorbing enough iron.

- Fatigue
- Unexplained bruising
- Bleeding from the nose, gums, rectum or other areas
- Sores in the mouth, on the tongue or rectum

With these symptoms, you could be suffering from aplastic anemia, a condition where your bone marrow does not produce enough blood cells. This is usually treatable, so see your doctor immediately.

- Headache
- Weakness
- Paleness
- Shortness of breath
- Confusion
- Depression
- Numbness and tingling in the arms and legs

You could be suffering from a vitamin B12 deficiency, also called pernicious anemia. Your body can't absorb vitamin B12, so the problem cannot be fixed by simple changes in your diet. You need to discuss it with your doctor.

- Redness on the tip and sides of your tongue, which later becomes bright red and swollen
- Fatigue
- Appetite loss
- Diarrhea and indigestion
- Headaches and backaches
- Sores on your skin
- Anxiety or confusion

If you aren't getting enough niacin, a B-complex vitamin, you may develop a disorder called pellagra. This is treatable with a balanced diet and niacin supplements. (See the *Food, vitamin, and mineral chart* on page 351.)

- Redness on the tip and sides of your tongue
- Contact with irritating foods or substances

You may be having a reaction to alcohol, tobacco products, spicy foods, mouthwashes, breath fresheners, or other items.

- You wear dentures

Correctly made and fitted dentures should not feel much different from your natural teeth. However, even the best dentist may not be able to get a perfect match every time. If your dentures rub or irritate your mouth, have your dentist recheck the fit.

265

> Small, painful sores on your tongue, lips, gums,
> throat, or inside your cheek

If you develop ulcers only on the inside of your
mouth, you probably are suffering from a common
ailment — canker sores.

Immediate help for canker sores

Canker sores affect anywhere from 20 to 50 percent of
the population, may be an inherited trait, and are more
common among women than men. Statistics show that if
you've had a canker sore before, you'll probably get one
again. Experts differ on the exact cause of these mouth
ulcers, but they do agree the condition is not caused by
a virus or bacteria, and is not contagious. The sores may
be a reaction to certain foods, emotional states like
fatigue and tension, or triggers like menstruation or
injury.

It begins as a small blister, which bursts and
becomes encircled by a bright red inflammation. It may
take up to two weeks for the sore to heal, which it usually does on its own. In the meantime, there are ways to
make yourself more comfortable and, perhaps, speed the
healing process.

* **Avoid irritating foods.** Tomatoes, citrus fruits,
  nuts, salsa, and chips are just some examples of
  foods that are salty, acidic, spicy, or abrasive.
  These can all aggravate canker sores. Stick to
  soft, bland food until the sores heal. Experts
  especially recommend yogurt.
* **Brush gently.** Don't scrub your gums, and avoid
  damaging the protective membrane that covers
  the sore.
* **Try some home-grown remedies.** Several homemade mouth rinses may coat the sores and relieve
  the pain. Try milk, milk of magnesia, or water
  with baking soda, salt, or hydrogen peroxide.
* **Visit your pharmacy.** Several over-the-counter
  ointments have numbing or waterproofing proper-
  ties to make you feel better and speed healing.
* **See your dentist.** A jagged tooth, braces, or dentures could be making your canker sore even

worse. Make sure there is no irritant in your mouth to prolong your discomfort.

The long-range plan for canker sores

If you frequently suffer from canker sores, visit your doctor. She can run blood and allergy tests to see if you have a preventable cause for the condition. A vitamin deficiency or food allergy is easy to fix.

Cold sores

It's one of life's little ironies. Just when you've got an important social event coming up, you feel that ominous tingle on your lip that means a cold sore is on its way. Don't cancel, and don't consider the paper-bag-over-the-head-trick. Try treating yourself with lysine to lessen the pain of cold sores and shorten their outbreak.

L-lysine is an amino acid you get through foods, like meat, cheese, milk, eggs, fish, beans, and potatoes, or through supplements you can buy at a health food store. To immediately treat a cold sore outbreak, experts recommend taking 3,000 milligrams (mg) of lysine each day until it's gone, then 500 mg daily to prevent it from coming back. If you take the supplements regularly, have your doctor monitor your cholesterol levels, since lysine may make your liver produce more cholesterol.

During an outbreak, you can make yourself more comfortable by eating popsicles or holding an ice cube to the sore, and staying away from salty or acidic foods. You also can apply over-the-counter and prescription ointments to numb the pain, reduce the chance of infection, and keep the sores from cracking.

Stress, colds or fever, menstruation, and sunlight are the most common triggers for a cold sore outbreak. Some of these are beyond your control, but others are not. Try to reduce the stress in your life, and apply an SPF 15 sunscreen to your lips for protection before going outside.

❖ **Practice good oral hygiene.** Gentle, thorough cleaning of your teeth and gums will keep your mouth healthy and in good shape to fight infection.

❖ **Take your prescription.** Your doctor may prescribe a treatment of antibiotics, such as tetracycline, or a prescription-strength topical anesthetic.

❖ **Gauge your emotions.** If you find that stress, anxiety, anger, or sadness brings on the canker sores, learn to control these feelings as much as possible. Your doctor can advise you of techniques and help groups.

Muscle cramps or weakness

Sudden intense pain in a muscle
Gradual weakening of muscles
General fatigue

Muscle cramps often are responsible for the aches and pains you feel all over your body. Anything from a "charley horse" or strained muscle to a serious sprain or tendinitis can cause your muscles to cramp or feel weak. Sometimes it's not something physical, but rather a chemical or mineral imbalance in your body that causes muscle problems. These are often symptoms of more serious conditions, such as dehydration or heat exhaustion.

Muscle weakness can also be a side effect of certain drugs or a nutritional deficiency. If you lack vitamin E, for example, you may find yourself feeling weak and unsteady. (See the *Food, vitamin, and mineral chart* on page 351.) Certain degenerative diseases, like muscular dystrophy or myasthenia gravis, also produce weak muscles. If you experience other symptoms as well, see your doctor.

⚕ It's time to see your doctor if you have muscle cramps or weakness and:

- Aches and cramping during exercise that stop when you rest
- Minor injuries that don't heal
- Chronic skin ulcerations
- Sudden onset of pain, coolness, and numbness in your leg

This could be intermittent claudication, a condition where your heart is unable to pump enough blood to your legs. It's a possible symptom of atherosclerosis, or hardening of the arteries, a serious artery disease that can lead to heart attack and stroke.

- Numbness in the arms and legs
- Paralyzed muscles in the face making swallowing difficult

You may have Guillain-Barré syndrome, a disease of the autoimmune system that usually follows a viral infection, such as flu, sore throat, or bronchitis.

- Confusion
- Pale skin
- Headache
- Fatigue
- Swelling

These symptoms suggest you may have too little or too much sodium in your blood. Since a sodium imbalance may signal an underlying disorder, see your doctor as soon as possible.

- Tingling or numbness in your hands and feet
- Seizures

These symptoms, along with an irregular heartbeat, may signal that you have too little calcium in your blood. This is a medical emergency, and you should get help immediately.

- Severe thirst
- Dry mouth and lips

- Little or no urine
- Sunken eyes
- Lightheadedness
- Rapid heart rate and breathing

These symptoms are a sign of dehydration, a common condition in older people. It can lead to more serious, sometimes fatal, conditions such as heat exhaustion and heatstroke.

- Weak, rapid pulse
- Cool, sweaty skin
- Dizziness
- Excessive thirst
- Nausea or vomiting

You may have heat exhaustion which means you've failed to drink enough fluids to replace body fluids and salt you've lost through sweating. Drink liquids and seek medical care immediately.

- Hot, dry skin
- Sudden faintness or dizziness
- High temperature
- Rapid heartbeat
- Headache and nausea
- Confusion

These are symptoms of heatstroke. Your body has overheated, and it reacts much like a car does — everything shuts down, including your brain. This is an emergency that requires immediate medical care.

Immediate help for heat exhaustion/heatstroke

Older people often suffer from heat-related illnesses because they sweat less and don't feel as thirsty as they used to. If you're exposed to hot temperatures for a long time, haven't been drinking enough fluids, or suffer a breakdown in your body's temperature mechanism, you may find yourself with heat exhaustion or heatstroke. Diabetes or heart disease increases your risk. If you don't get immediate medical attention, your body will

Keeping your electrolytes balanced

Water is one of your most important nutrients when it comes to preventing muscle cramps and weakness. It plays a key role in maintaining balance inside your body because it's the one nutrient that can slip freely back and forth across cell walls.

To prevent too much or too little water from entering your cells, your body uses electrolytes to move fluids around and keep them where they're supposed to be.

These electrolytes are formed when mineral salts in your body dissolve into single particles that carry an electrical current. Water will flow to an area that has more of these particles, so wherever your cells tell the electrolytes to go, water will follow.

Your body uses several methods to regulate water intake and maintain fluid and electrolyte balance, such as the thirst mechanism. When your blood has too much salt and other minerals, it "borrows" water from your salivary glands, making you feel thirsty.

Your brain center, known as the hypothalamus, monitors your blood concentration and signals when it's time for a drink, but sometimes the signal comes too late.

Your body has another control, antidiuretic hormone (ADH), which regulates your kidneys. This helps ensure your body only excretes water it doesn't need.

When your body is dehydrated, particularly from vomiting or diarrhea, it panics and starts pulling water from cells in every part of your body. This can disrupt your heart and eventually cause death if you don't replace your body's minerals and water.

shut down completely. About half the elderly who suffer from this serious problem will die without treatment.

If you experience any symptoms of excessive heat, stop what you're doing, get something to drink, find shade, and ask for help.

❖ **Cool rapidly.** A heatstroke victim will be extremely hot but not sweating. You should move him to a cool place; wrap him in wet sheets, if necessary; and get him to a hospital immediately.

❖ **Drink liquids.** If the person feels faint but is sweating, that's a sign of heat exhaustion. Try giving him some fluids, such as water or juice, and then take him to a medical center.

❖ **Avoid self-medicating.** Don't take salt pills to try to replace your lost sodium. Leave it to medical personnel to determine what you need to restore your body's chemical balance.

The long-range plan for heat exhaustion/heatstroke

Heavy sweating, vomiting, or diarrhea can lead to dehydration if you don't replace the fluids you lose. These conditions are especially dangerous because they flush away your body's much-needed supply of salt. And, of course, dehydration can lead to even more serious problems like heatstroke, heat exhaustion, or hypothermia (loss of body heat). These conditions are easy to avoid by taking the proper precautions.

❖ **Lighten up on clothing.** Wear light, loose-fitting styles when you're out in hot weather. Make sure your body is not constricted. Tight-fitting clothes make it harder for your sweat to evaporate, and sweating is your body's most effective way to cool down. Lighter colors also feel cooler since they don't absorb the heat as much as dark colors.

❖ **Fan that breeze.** Keep yourself cool whenever possible. If you do get overheated, sit in front of a fan, air conditioner, or even a window and enjoy a cool breeze.

❖ **Beware of hot tubs.** You may love to relax away your cares in a hot tub or sauna, but these settings pose a health risk if you're not careful. Heat-associated deaths have been linked to saunas, hot tubs, and whirlpool baths. Limit your time, and get out immediately if you feel lightheaded or ill in any way.

❖ **Drink, drink, drink!** Don't wait until you're thirsty to have some water. Keep a water bottle handy and sip it throughout the day. Your thirst mechanism often doesn't kick in until you're already low on fluids. Drink extra water if you tend to sweat heavily.

Nausea and vomiting

An uncomfortable, unsettled feeling in your stomach
Uncontrollable loss of your stomach contents
through your mouth

You have a queasy feeling in the pit of your stomach. That might make you happy if you're a young woman trying to have a baby. But most people would just as soon avoid the feeling, and they probably could do without the upheaval of vomiting. Nausea and vomiting can result from a temporary stomach virus, a medicine you are taking, or something more serious and rare, like stomach cancer or a severe head injury.

 It's time to see your doctor if you have nausea/vomiting and:

Fever
Neck stiffness
Headache
Sensitivity to light

If you have these symptoms, you may have meningitis, which is an infection of the spinal fluid and the tissues around the brain and spinal cord.

Loss of appetite
Stomach pain
Mild fever
Severe constipation

If your abdominal pain is relieved by drawing your right thigh up while lying still, and you have the above symptoms, you may have appendicitis.

- Abdominal pain
- Mild fever
- Abdominal bloating
- Mild jaundice (a yellow tint to the skin)

These symptoms may indicate you have pancreatitis, which is an inflammation of your pancreas.

- Stomach pain
- Gas and bloating
- Jaundice (a yellow tint to the skin)
- Indigestion after eating fatty foods

You may have gallstones, especially if the pain is in your upper right abdomen or between your shoulder blades. Gallstones are hard crystals, usually made up of cholesterol, which form in your gallbladder. (See also *Belching, bloating, and gas* chapter.)

- Ringing in your ears
- Headache
- Feel dizzy, weak, or confused
- Chest pain

If you have these symptoms, carbon monoxide poisoning may be the problem. Car exhaust and faulty heaters are common causes of carbon monoxide poisoning. (See also *Headache* chapter.)

- Vomiting
- Stomach pain
- Diarrhea (sometimes bloody)
- Other people who ate the same food also get sick

If you experience these problems after eating a meal, you may have a form of food poisoning. Depending on the type of poison, you may feel sick as early as one hour after eating contaminated food or as long as three to five days after. Though most cases of food poisoning will run their course without serious complications, severe cases should be treated by a doctor. (See also *Abdominal pain, sudden* chapter.)

- **Heavy sweating**
- **Dizziness**
- **Paleness**
- **Feel tired, weak, or confused**

If you have these symptoms, especially if you have been in a moving vehicle, you probably have motion sickness.

Immediate help for motion sickness

You go deep sea fishing and spend more time reeling with nausea than reeling in fish. You spend airplane flights clutching a little plastic bag protectively to your chest. You have motion sickness, but don't worry. It's not really a sickness at all, although it certainly makes you feel sick.

Motion sickness is actually a normal response to abnormal movement. You have a balance center in your inner ear that gets confused when the motion you feel doesn't match what your eyes see. That's why a fast-moving video game can make you sick, because your eye sees the screen moving quickly, but your body is sitting still. This confusion can give you a headache and slight queasiness, or you may find yourself sweating heavily, turning pale, and possibly vomiting.

The best way to deal with motion sickness is simply to stop what you are doing. If you are on a car trip, pull off the road for a few minutes and sit with your eyes closed. On an airplane, take slow deep breaths and try to remain calm. Being anxious and tense will only make your motion sickness worse.

Believe it or not, acupressure may help ease your queasiness as well. Hold your hand with your palm up. Find the spot on your forearm that is three finger widths from your wrist, between the two tendons and lined up with your middle finger. Apply steady pressure to this point, and you may soon begin to feel your motion sickness fade away.

275

Though these tips may make you feel better, the best way to deal with motion sickness is to prevent it in the first place.

The long-range plan for motion sickness

If you have this problem, you may not look forward to vacations as much as the rest of your family. Don't put a damper on everyone's fun by refusing to get on that plane, train, or automobile. Instead, use these tips to nip the problem in the bud.

- ❖ **Keep it fresh.** Certain heavy odors, like cigarette smoke, can make your motion sickness worse. Try to keep the air you breathe fresh and scent-free.
- ❖ **Get it in focus.** You feel sick because your eyes and your inner ear don't agree. It sometimes helps to focus on the horizon or some other object to make yourself believe you're seeing and feeling the same motion.
- ❖ **Rest before you go.** Make sure you get plenty of rest before embarking on any trip that may cause motion sickness.
- ❖ **Axe the alcohol.** Pass on any alcoholic beverages both before and during your trip.
- ❖ **Keep it light.** Large heavy meals can distress your stomach and make motion sickness more likely. Try to eat small meals, and avoid fatty foods.
- ❖ **Get some ginger.** Studies find that ginger can tone down your nausea and help prevent vomiting, although it may not help with other symptoms, like headache and dizziness. One study looked at people who took a 940-milligram capsule of ginger before spinning in a chair. They were less likely to vomit than people who took Dramamine, which is a medicine for preventing motion sickness. You can find ginger in different forms at your health food store, or try sipping the original nausea-buster, ginger ale. But stick to health store brands; supermarket ginger ale usually doesn't contain enough ginger to help.
- ❖ **Behavior therapy may help.** Imagine being a sailor, truck driver, or flight attendant fighting the misery

of motion sickness. If your job exposes you to motion all the time, behavior therapy may help. You can call your local counseling center to see if it offers this type of therapy. But keep in mind that therapy usually takes a long time and may not be the best solution for occasional motion sickness.

If you love sailing, despite your queasy stomach, don't give up yet. This type of sickness tends to get better if you keep experiencing the motion that bothers you. Just follow the above tips and tough it out. Chances are, your motion sickness will disappear soon, and you'll enjoy smooth sailing from now on.

Neck pain

Discomfort, soreness, or stiffness in your neck

The seven vertebrae at the top of your backbone, called the cervical spine, are made up of alternating layers of bone and soft cartilage, with nerves and the spinal cord running through the middle. This is, basically, your neck, which holds your head up, allows it to move, and links it to the rest of your body. Your neck must be extremely flexible in order to do all the things you ask of it. Things like looking over your shoulder before passing on the highway, gazing up at the stars, and checking to see if your belt is buckled. Your neck is, however, quite unprotected. That, along with its curved construction, makes it particularly vulnerable to injury. If you are experiencing neck pain, and you think it's more than a simple muscle strain, see your doctor.

⚕ It's time to see your doctor if you have neck pain and:

- A recent injury
- Dizziness

- Headache
- Nausea

If you are experiencing these symptoms and have fallen or have been in a car, diving, or sports-related accident, you need immediate medical care. You may have fractured your neck or be suffering from whiplash, a forced violent backward or forward motion of your neck muscles.

- **Difficulty in moving an arm or leg**
- **Loss of bladder or bowel control**
- **Back pain**

If you've recently had a fall or injury and have these symptoms, don't move. Get someone to call your doctor. You may have a spinal cord injury.

- **A sudden sharp pain down the back of your leg**
- **Numbness or tingling in an arm or leg**
- **Back pain**

Pain, numbness, or tingling in an arm or leg, especially with back or neck pain, may mean pressure or damage to your spine from a ruptured disk. (See also **Back pain** chapter.)

- **Fever**
- **Neck stiffness**
- **Nausea and vomiting**
- **Sensitivity to light**
- **Headache**
- **Fatigue**

If you have these symptoms, you may have meningitis, which is an infection of the spinal fluid and the tissues around the brain and spinal cord.

- **Fever**
- **Headache**
- **Vomiting**
- **Neck and back stiffness**

These are only the first mild symptoms of a viral disease of the brain called encephalitis. More severe cases may cause seizures and coma.

- A stiff neck and dizziness when you turn your head
- Pain that extends to your shoulders and arms
- Weakness and loss of sensation in your fingers, hands, and arms

These symptoms point to cervical spondylosis, which is pressure on the nerves in your neck caused by arthritis or the deterioration of the bones in your neck. See your doctor for help in managing this condition.

- Morning neck stiffness
- Limited movement and dexterity

This could mean osteoarthritis, a condition where the cartilage in your joints gradually breaks down. Usually, you will feel an aching pain when you move or put weight on your joints. (See also *Knee pain* chapter.)

- Swelling and redness in your neck
- Low fever
- General ill-feeling
- Severe morning stiffness that can last for hours

These symptoms may indicate the onset of rheumatoid arthritis, a disease that inflames the joints.

- Neck stiffness
- Achiness, especially in the morning
- Restricted movement of the joint

Approximately 37 million Americans suffer from arthritis, which means inflammation of a joint. It can be caused by more than 100 different diseases and, in most cases, has no cure. By adjusting your lifestyle and taking responsibility for managing your pain, you can lead a normal, productive life. (See also *Joint pain* chapter.)

- Painful muscle spasms in your neck
- Shortened neck muscles that cause your head to twist sideways and down

Torticollis, or wryneck, as it is sometimes called, can be periodic or permanent. This condition is usually the result of either an injury to or inflammation of the neck muscles, although stress and emotional problems can also be a factor.

- Dull ache in your neck
- Neck stiffness
- Pain with movement into certain positions
- Headache or dizziness
- Referred pain in your shoulder or arm

These symptoms indicate a fairly straightforward condition — a muscle strain. Usually this happens after a particular activity or as a result of forcing your neck into an unnatural position.

Immediate help for neck strain

If you wake one morning with a stiff neck and find yourself suffering from pain throughout the day, first eliminate any of the more serious problems listed above. If you feel confident that you don't have a critical condition, you may be suffering from a simple muscle strain. Even though a muscle strain can be painful, it is not life-threatening. Here are some tips to help you recover more quickly.

- ❖ **Warm it up.** Moist heat applied to your neck, back, and shoulders will reduce your pain and loosen up your muscles. You might want to take a few moments with a heating pad before you start any therapeutic exercises.

- ❖ **Massage it out.** Whether you go to a professional masseuse or simply enlist a family member into the job, a rubdown on your neck, shoulders, and upper back will feel heavenly and relax tense or spasmed muscles at the same time.

- ❖ **Punch the nighttime clock.** Stress and fatigue are a lethal combination for your body, so make sure you are getting not only the proper amount of sleep, but the proper kind of sleep, as well. Leave the day's worries behind as you climb into bed for a deep, restful sleep.

Exercises to relieve a sore neck

❖ Sit or stand comfortably. Pull your chin into your neck without lifting it. Breathe in and push your shoulders back and up. Hold for a few seconds, then relax.

❖ Retract your chin, then slowly let your head drop back as far as comfortable. With shoulders relaxed, slowly roll your head slightly to the left, then the right. Continue with about six of these small movements, then pull your head back up.

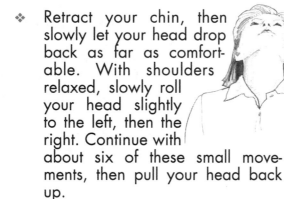

❖ Retract your chin and stretch your neck sideways by lowering your ear toward your shoulder. Repeat on the other side.

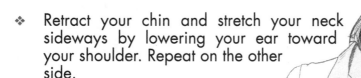

❖ Retract your chin and, keeping your head level, slowly swing your chin around to first one shoulder then the other.

The long-range plan for neck strain

You must make some definite changes in your habits if you want to avoid further neck strain.

❖ **Practice positive posture.** The way you sit and stand has a tremendous influence on every joint in your body. In order to be kind to your neck, you must first realize the stress poor posture places on it. Freeze for a moment and examine your posture right now. Are you sitting slumped in a chair, leaning over a table, propped up in bed, or on the sofa with your neck against the arm? All of these positions may feel comfortable at first, but they put your neck and back at an awkward angle. Chances are, when you get up, you're going to feel an ache in those muscles. If you continually sit or lie with your head forced one way or another, you are asking for a stiff neck that really is a pain.

To keep yourself sitting tall, scoot your bottom all the way to the back of your chair and place a small pillow in the hollow of your lower back. Don't jut your chin up or out — keep it tucked in. Choose a chair with arms. This will give your back, shoulders, and neck additional support.

❖ **Don't sleep like a baby.** Unlike infants who can curl up anywhere and never feel the consequences, you must examine your sleeping positions and your pillow. These are two major culprits of sore necks. Don't sleep on your stomach, since this forces your neck to one side or the other. If you sleep on your back, make sure your pillow is not too high. The best size keeps your neck parallel with the bed. As a side sleeper, you may have the hardest time keeping your neck straight. It is very important to align your head with your spine. Try one of the orthopedic pillows that are on the market. Never sleep in a chair or slumped across a couch.

❖ **Adjust your activities.**
  ● If you spend your day at a desk or table, make sure your chair is the right height to keep you from bending or leaning.

Exercises to strengthen neck muscles

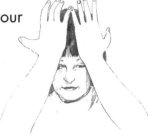

❖ Place the palms of your hands on your forehead. Push your head into your hands while resisting the motion with your palms. Hold for about two seconds. Repeat five times.

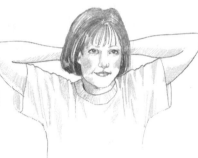

❖ Lock your fingers and place them behind your head. Push backward against your hands. Your head should not move. Hold for about two seconds and repeat five times.

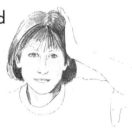

❖ Place your right palm against your head just above your right ear. Push against your hand, resisting the motion with your hand. Hold for about two seconds. Repeat five times on each side.

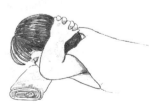

❖ Lie on your stomach with a small towel under your forehead. Lock your fingers behind your head. Slowly lift your shoulders and head slightly. Lower back to the floor and repeat five times.

- Have a small step stool handy for those top shelves in the kitchen or garage. Reaching up can be just as harmful as bending down.
- Bifocals are a fact of life for most older adults, and it is easy to get into that bad habit of shifting your neck up and down to see properly. Try to lift your book or paper to the proper angle and save your neck.
- Don't cradle the telephone receiver between your neck and your ear. This places a terrible strain on your neck muscles. Add a foam attachment to the handset if you can't break the habit.
- Take a moment before driving off to check your car seat. Is it too far back? Do you need to sit on a cushion? Tilt the steering wheel, if necessary, to keep your shoulders at a good angle.

Nose, runny or stuffy

A drippy, runny nose
A stuffy nose that makes breathing difficult

Babies and young children are always adorable, runny noses and all. In adults, however, a loud sniff or snort from a runny or stuffy nose is considerably less appealing. A nasal problem isn't life-threatening, but it is uncomfortable and annoying. Occasionally, a runny or stuffy nose signals a situation in which you may need your doctor's help.

⚕ It's time to see your doctor if you have a runny or stuffy nose and:

- The feeling that air is not flowing freely through your nose
- Chronic colds or sinus infections

- A crooked nose, or an injury to your nose in the
     past

These are the signs of a deviated septum, which
means the ridge of cartilage and bone running
down the center of your nose is crooked, either
from injury or because it simply grew that way.
This causes problems with the air flow in your
nose, which means you may have more colds and
sinus infections. Surgery can correct the problem.

- Sinus drainage
- Headache
- Pain around your eyes and cheeks
- Bad breath
- A general ill feeling

Along with these symptoms, a constant runny nose
may signal a sinus infection or inflammation,
called sinusitis.

- A sense of smell that is not as strong as it used to be
- The feeling that air is not flowing freely through
     your nose
- Pain and a heavy feeling in your face and nose

These symptoms could indicate a condition called
nasal polyps, fluid-filled sacs that grow in your
sinuses. They are not cancerous or dangerous, but
they are uncomfortable and make breathing
through your nose difficult. Your doctor can
remove them through minor surgery.

- Itchy, watery eyes
- Itchy nose and scratchy throat
- Sneezing
- Fatigue
- Dark circles under your eyes

Along with a runny or stuffy nose, these are the
symptoms of allergic rhinitis, commonly known as
"allergy." It's usually caused by your body's reaction
to pollen, dust mites, mold, or animals. If your allergy is severe and really making you uncomfortable,
your doctor can probably give you medicine to help
you feel better. (See also *Eye problems* chapter.)

- Headache
- Cough
- Sore throat
- Fever and chills
- Aching muscles
- Fatigue

If you have these symptoms along with your runny nose, you probably have influenza, or "flu," a common respiratory infection. It's caused by a virus and is contagious.

Immediate help for colds and flu

If you don't have the achy muscles, headache, and extreme fatigue of the flu, consider yourself lucky. If you do have a runny or stuffy nose, sore throat, watery eyes, cough, and low-grade fever, you probably have the most common illness in the world — a cold. Like the flu, a cold is caused by a virus, but it's less serious. Most people get over the flu in about a week, but it can be life-threatening for certain people, such as babies, the elderly, and those with chronic illnesses.

Even though a cold and the flu are quite different, they share some symptoms. They also share some treatments for home-care.

❖ **Stay fluid.** Drinking plenty of liquid is important to keep your body functioning well at any time, but it's especially important when you have a cold or the flu. If you have a fever, you need extra liquid to keep from dehydrating. It also helps thin secretions from your lungs so you can cough them up. Eight to 10 cups of liquid a day should do it. Most people find hot drinks more soothing than cold ones.

❖ **Gargle.** The best and most comforting gargle for your sore throat is warm, salty water. One-half teaspoon stirred into a cup of warm water will make a soothing solution. Another good gargle is strong, brewed tea, which has an astringent, or drying, effect. You can drink it warm or cold.

❖ **Rest easy.** When your body is working to fight off a cold or the flu, it needs plenty of extra rest. Don't push yourself when you don't feel like it. If you have the flu, you don't have much choice — you have to rest. Even if you just have a bad cold, a day off from your normal activities will be good for your health in the long run. And it might protect your friends and co-workers from catching your germs.

❖ **Investigate echinacea.** This interesting herb helps stimulate your body's own defenses against bacteria and viruses. If you take it early in the course of a cold, your illness may be shorter and less severe. Echinacea comes in liquid or tablet form and is available in most stores that sell herbal remedies.

❖ **Steam it up.** Hot, moist air can temporarily clear stuffy nasal passages and make you feel better. Take a hot shower or use a humidifier. Or you can make your own temporary humidifier. Simply boil a pot of fresh water, put it on a table, then lean over the pot with a towel over your head, and breathe deeply. If you add the sweet-smelling herb chamomile to the hot water, you'll reap even more benefits from the fragrant steam. Chamomile has the ability to help clear clogged sinuses and soothe an irritated throat.

❖ **Keep your nose clean.** A nasal wash, or nasal irrigation, is an excellent tool for fighting a cold or the flu. It washes bacteria and excess mucus from your sinuses and helps prevent a sinus infection. You'll need a large rubber syringe that you can buy at your local drugstore.

Make a solution of one-half teaspoon of plain (not iodized) salt and a pinch of baking soda mixed with one cup of warm water. Fill the syringe, then place it in one nostril and pinch the nostril closed around it. Squeeze the syringe to move the saline solution through your nose, then blow your nose gently. Most of the salty solution will come out through your mouth, so just rinse with plain water to remove it. Continue until the drainage is clean, then repeat with the other nostril. To keep

Sinusitis self-defense

Pressure, pain, and swelling in your face could mean your sinuses are inflamed. Fight back with these tips:

❖ **Look for an allergy.** Your sinus problems could be caused by hay fever or something else in your environment. Keep track of when and where sinusitis strikes. You may be able to pinpoint and eliminate the cause.

❖ **Use a vaporizer.** Warm, moist air will help your sinuses drain.

❖ **Drink plenty of liquids.** Eight to 10 glasses of fluid a day is a good rule of thumb. It will help thin the mucus and clear your nasal passages.

❖ **Raise your head when you sleep.** Put extra pillows under your head so mucus won't drain back into your sinuses. If sinus pressure is worse on one side, sleep on the other side.

❖ **Go for the burn.** Eating hot, spicy foods or herbs, such as hot chiles, horseradish, or garlic, will help open your nasal passages.

❖ **Wash it out.** A nasal wash using warm salt water and a rubber syringe can be a huge help in treating and preventing sinusitis.

❖ **Spray it away.** An over-the-counter nasal spray can give you relief, but don't use it more than three days. Your doctor may prescribe a corticosteroid spray that will reduce inflammation in your nose. It may take several weeks to get results, but it can really help sinus drainage.

❖ **Antibiotics may help.** If the discharge from your stuffy nose turns greenish-yellow, it's time to see your doctor.

your nasal syringe from reinfecting you later, be sure to clean it well after every use. Store it on end in a clean glass so any remaining water can drain out, and make sure every family member has his own syringe.

❖ **Zap it with zinc.** Researchers have found that zinc gluconate may be an effective weapon in the war against colds. In scientific studies, people who used zinc gluconate lozenges while they had a cold got well twice as fast as those who didn't use them. Zinc lozenges are now available over the counter. You may find they taste bitter, even though they have fruit flavoring added. But if you really want to get over your cold quickly, zinc gluconate lozenges might be worth a try.

❖ **Discard the dirties.** With a cold or flu, you'll probably blow your nose a lot. Be sure to use disposable tissues instead of handkerchiefs. Then you won't reinfect yourself as you're getting well, and you're less likely to infect others. Dispose of dirty tissues carefully in a sealed bag.

❖ **Soothe your aching back.** To comfort your aching back and muscles, try a heating pad or warm compress. You can make a quick compress from a towel soaked in hot water and wrung out.

The long-range plan for colds and flu

The best approach to treating colds and flu is to avoid getting them in the first place. Here are some steps you can take to keep a vicious virus out of your life.

❖ **Celebrate C.** Not all scientists agree about the value of vitamin C in fighting a cold or other infection. But some studies have shown that it can make cold symptoms milder and chase the cold away sooner. It also may prevent colds in the first place. So, boost your overall health and resistance to infection with a diet that includes plenty of vitamin C in the form of fresh fruits and vegetables. (See the *Food, vitamin, and mineral chart* on page 351.)

❖ **Stave off stress.** When you're under stress, your immune system doesn't work as well as it should.

This makes your body more vulnerable to infections, including colds and flu. Try to get a handle on your problems by keeping your sense of humor and a healthy perspective. Eliminate the unimportant things in your life. Make time for the people and activities you really care about.

❖ **Keep those hands clean.** If you've been shopping, cashing a check, attending a baseball game, or doing anything else in a public place, wash your hands when you get home. Thousands of people with dirty, germy hands have touched the same door handles, stair rails, elevator buttons, and money. You pick up their bacteria and viruses and infect yourself when you touch your eyes, mouth, or the food you eat.

The best soap to get rid of germs is liquid antibacterial hand soap in a pump bottle. Bar soap can actually harbor cold germs on its surface. It's easy and inexpensive to take along little packets of antibacterial towelettes to wash your hands before a meal or anytime you've been somewhere especially dirty. It's a simple thing, but it could determine whether you catch a cold or the flu.

❖ **Make a clean sweep.** Keep your house really clean and germ-free, and you'll protect yourself from colds and flu. Use an antibacterial cleanser, or a solution of bleach and water, to clean kitchen counters, doorknobs, cabinet handles, staircase railings, telephones, and anything else you touch often.

Let your dishes air dry, or dry them in the dishwasher. Don't use a dish towel; it provides a warm environment for bacteria. Frequently change the dishcloth you use to clean kitchen counters. It could become a germ factory if it's left wet for long. If you use a sponge, try the new antibacterial kind, and throw it out if it gets too dirty. Both sponges and dish brushes can be washed in the dishwasher to give them a clean, new start. You may feel like you're going overboard, but that extra cleaning could knock out a stray virus that would give you or your family a bad cold or case of the flu.

❖ **Give up smoking.** Cigarette smoke can lower your resistance to disease, whether you're the person smoking or breathing the smoke secondhand. If you smoke and get a cold, it's more likely to turn into something worse like bronchitis. Nicotine gum and patches are available at any drugstore today to help you beat this habit. Do yourself and the people around you a favor, and give it up.

❖ **Get a flu shot.** Do you have diabetes; heart disease; lung, kidney, or blood problems; asthma; or an immune system that doesn't work well? Are you elderly or undergoing chemotherapy? If so, you should probably have a flu shot. All these conditions put you at higher risk of getting the flu, and a vaccination can probably prevent it.

Based on research and statistics, scientists create a new vaccine every year, including the A and B viruses they think will be around the next winter. Sometimes a new, unknown strain will surface. But if you've had the flu vaccine, even this new flu shouldn't hit you as hard.

Fall is the best time of year to get a flu shot, from October through November. This is six to eight weeks before the flu season starts. It takes a while for your body to produce antibodies, its ammunition against the virus. The most common side effect of a vaccination is a sore spot on your arm from the shot. Some people may have fever, sore muscles, and fatigue for a couple of days after the vaccination, but not a full-blown case of the flu. If you're allergic to eggs, don't get a flu vaccine. It may contain a small amount of egg protein.

❖ **Avoid antihistamines.** These medicines block histamine, a chemical released in your body when it reacts to such things as pollen and dust. Antihistamines are excellent for allergy and hay fever, but not as helpful for a cold.

Scientists have finally come up with a flu medicine that really works, although it only fights influenza type A. If you take rimantadine within 48 hours after your illness begins, you should have shorter and less severe symptoms. This is a real help if you haven't had a flu vaccine.

For a cure to the common cold, you'll have to wait a little longer. Recently, scientists have seen some promising results on experiments with cold viruses. But successfully beating the army of cold germs in the world is an ongoing battle. Until that war is won, use our treatment tips to make yourself comfortable, and try to avoid the problem as much as you can.

The hazards of antibiotics

When something is broken, you want it fixed. And if you have a cold, you want something to make it go away. That's fine, unless your doctor automatically prescribes an antibiotic.

The common cold is caused by a virus, not bacteria. So unless you have a bacterial infection along with your cold, an antibiotic isn't going to do you any good, and it could actually do some harm.

Today, new strains of bacteria have developed that resist antibiotic treatment. This is partly because doctors prescribe the medicines too often for minor illnesses such as colds. Another problem is that people don't always take the entire amount of medicine that's prescribed.

If you take the medicine only until you feel better, the bacteria are not killed off. They often bounce back in a new resistant form. You may pass this "super" bacteria on to someone else, but the old antibiotic will no longer work. New types of antibiotics, called "wide spectrum," are used against the new, resistant strains; but they're not always successful. And when they're used improperly, more drug-resistant strains develop.

So what's a person to do? Don't take an antibiotic unless your doctor says you have a bacterial infection along with your cold. If he does give you a prescription, take all of it, even if you already feel much better before you run out of medicine.

Rectal problems

Pain, bleeding, or itching in the rectal area

There is nothing that can quite match rectal discomfort. Whether you have an itch you can't scratch, bleeding you don't understand, or pain that makes every chair seem to grow thorns, all you really want is relief. This is one situation where consulting an expert is the fastest route to peace of mind.

 ## It's time to see your doctor if you have:

- Rectal bleeding
- Fatigue
- Bleeding from the nose, gums, or other areas
- Sores in your mouth or on your tongue or rectum
- Unexplained bruising

With these symptoms, you could be suffering from aplastic anemia, a condition where your bone marrow does not produce enough blood cells. This is usually treatable, so see your doctor immediately.

- Rectal pain
- Blood or mucous discharge from rectum
- Abdominal cramping on your lower left side
- Constipation

These symptoms could mean you have proctitis, which is an inflammation of the rectum and the area around the anus.

- Rectal bleeding or blood in your stool
- Cramping abdominal pain
- Fever or nausea
- Tenderness in area over colon

If you have any of these symptoms, you may have diverticulitis, an infection or inflammation of small pouches that can form in the walls of your intestine. (See also *Abdominal pain, frequent* chapter.)

- Rectal bleeding or blood in your stool
- A recurrent, burning-type pain in your upper abdomen lasting 30 minutes to three hours
- Unexplained change in appetite or weight
- Vomiting

If you have this combination of symptoms, you may have an ulcer. Ulcers are small sores in the lining of your stomach or intestines. Although many people still think stress causes ulcers, tiny spiral-shaped bacteria called *Helicobacter pylori (H. pylori)* are considered to be the main cause. (See also *Abdominal pain, frequent* chapter.)

- Itching around the anus and genitals

A variety of things can cause this condition, but the most common are contact dermatitis, psoriasis, chronic diarrhea, tight clothing, and yeast infections.

- Rectal bleeding
- Rectal pain during hard bowel movement
- Rectal itching
- Muscle spasms (sometimes)

If you notice blood on the toilet paper after a large, hard stool, you have probably torn or split the skin around your anus. This is called an anal fissure. Consult your doctor for treatment of frequent or constant fissures.

- Occasional sharp rectal pain lasting several seconds to several minutes, most often occurring at night
- An urge to defecate, but pain and difficulty doing so
- Relief of pain with a bowel movement or orgasm (sometimes)

Proctalgia fugax is a common but little diagnosed condition that experts believe is caused by either a muscle or blood vessel spasm.

- Rectal pain and cramping
- Bloody diarrhea
- Left abdominal pain
- Nausea and appetite loss
- Fever

These symptoms could be due to ulcerative colitis, a serious colon disease with no known cause.

- Rectal bleeding, pain, and itching
- Mucous discharge from rectum
- Small bulge around anus

These symptoms indicate hemorrhoids, which are swollen veins in the anus or rectum.

- Change in bowel movements (diarrhea or constipation)
- Blood in the stool or rectal bleeding
- Rectal or abdominal pain
- A feeling of pressure on the rectum

If you experience these symptoms, you should discuss with your doctor the possibility of colorectal cancer, which is cancer in your colon and/or rectum.

5 ways to relieve painful hemorrhoids

❖ **Sitz down.** A soak in a few inches of warm water for around 10 minutes, several times a day, will really ease your pain. Relax in your tub or you can find Sitz Baths at your local pharmacy, very reasonably priced.

❖ **Cool the heat.** If your hemorrhoids are painfully swollen, take this as an excuse to rest. Stay in bed for a few hours with an ice pack on your anal area.

❖ **Grab a footstool.** Prop your feet up at least a few inches during bowel movements to prevent straining.

❖ **Clean well, but gently.** Use soft, moist tissues to wipe after a bowel movement.

Immediate help for colorectal cancer

Cancer of the colon and rectum kills 60,000 people each year, making it the third highest deadly cancer in the United States. This is particularly tragic since early treatment can cure 70 to 90 percent of colorectal cancers. If you are over 40; have a family history of colon or colorectal cancer; suffer from other colon or bowel disorders, such as irritable bowel syndrome, colon polyps, or

Lifestyle changes help control hemorrhoids

❖ **Don't hurry, but ...** Straining during a bowel movement is one of the major causes of hemorrhoids. So, don't rush the process, but don't sit too long either. It's better to become regular through other changes, not force.

❖ **Adjust your diet.** Any doctor you see will discuss diet as a way of improving this condition. Lots of fiber from bran, fruits, vegetables, and whole grains will soften the stool and relieve the pressure on your hemorrhoids.

❖ **Drink, drink, drink, drink.** And it doesn't have to be just water, although it's hard to beat water's health benefits. As long as you are getting six to eight glasses of liquid each day, you are flushing out your digestive system. Stay away from alcohol, though, as this will actually dehydrate you.

❖ **Stay active.** Hemorrhoids should not restrict your normal exercise routine. In fact, it is more important than ever for you to keep your body fit. Regular physical activity will improve your bowel function.

❖ **Slim down.** Being overweight is often a consequence of an inactive lifestyle and poor diet. Changing these two aspects of your life will not only improve your overall health and the condition of your hemorrhoids, but reduce the force of excess weight on your body.

colitis; or have a diet high in animal fat and low in fiber, you have a greater risk of developing colorectal cancer.

❖ **Conduct a home test.** If you are in the high risk category for developing colorectal cancer, experts recommend testing your stool for blood at least every two years. Your doctor can provide you with a test kit and instructions. Make sure you understand and follow them exactly. Studies show this method of early detection reduces colorectal cancer deaths significantly.

The long-range plan for colorectal cancer

Regular checkups with your doctor are one of your best detection tools, but there are several dietary adjustments you can make to aid you in your fight against colorectal cancer.

❖ **Increase your calcium.** Vitamin D-fortified calcium products seem to inhibit colon cancer, perhaps by protecting the lining of your colon

❖ **Increase your water-insoluble fiber.** This kind of fiber will not dissolve in water, which is helpful in speeding the movement of cancer-causing elements through your colon. Foods such as brown rice, legumes, seeds, wheat bran, and whole grains are high in water-insoluble fiber.

❖ **Eat your vegetables.** Crucifer vegetables, like cabbage, broccoli, watercress, white and red radishes, cauliflower, and brussels sprouts, increase the amount of tumor-inhibiting enzymes your body produces.

❖ **Pick a fruit.** Apples, pears, strawberries, plums, and tangerines are high in pectin, a fruit fiber that's even better for you than bran.

❖ **Add an amino acid.** Methionine is a nutrient that battles colon cancer. It is found in sunflower seeds, wheat germ, oat flakes, granola, cheese, milk, and eggs.

❖ **Take an aspirin, or two, or three.** A recent medical study shows it takes 10 years of regular aspirin use (four to six tablets per week) to significantly reduce your risk of colorectal cancer. Consult your doctor.

❖ **Avoid a high fat, high protein, low fiber diet.** All these food components work against your body's natural cancer defenses. For example, a diet high in fat sets a perfect environment for the development of cancer by increasing the amount of bile acids in your colon. These bile acids, which are necessary for the digestion of fats, promote tumors. It would be impossible to list all foods and their impact on colorectal cancer, but you can make sensible decisions based on a couple of guidelines. First, divide foods into two groups: animal products and plant products. Within the animal product group, you have meat and dairy products, which contain protein and other nutrients as well as fat. Fruits, vegetables, and grain products are highest in fiber and vitamins. Of course, there are healthy and unhealthy food selections within all groups, but usually the more natural the food is, the healthier it is for you.

Sexual pain

Pain or discomfort in the genitals when having sexual intercourse

For most couples, sexual intimacy is a warm and special part of a loving marriage, and it can last throughout your lives together. As you age, you may have to make allowances for physical limitations that affect your sex life. But when sex becomes downright painful, it can cast a cold chill over even the warmest of relationships. The problem is most likely a minor one, but sexual pain can indicate a more serious problem that needs the attention of your doctor.

 For men, it's time to see your doctor if you have sexual pain and:

> An erection that is painful and tender, continues
> too long, and is not caused by sexual arousal

This is an emergency situation called priapism and you should seek medical help immediately.

> Blisters or sores on the skin of your penis, or red-
> ness and painful swelling
> Swollen lymph glands in your groin

This may indicate an infection or inflammation of your skin such as genital herpes, which is a viral infection; or balanitis, an inflammation due to bacterial or fungal infection; or an allergic reaction.

> Frequent, burning urination
> Problems in beginning the urine stream and emp-
> tying your bladder
> Fever and chills
> Low back pain
> Achy muscles and joints
> Unusual discharge from your penis

These symptoms could point to an infection of your prostate gland, known as prostatitis; a sexually transmitted disease such as gonorrhea; or an infection of your urethra, the tube that carries urine from your bladder.

Immediate help for prostatitis

If your doctor diagnoses your problem as a prostate infection, he may prescribe an antibiotic to fight it, along with something for your pain and a stool softener to keep you from getting constipated. It's important to get treatment and avoid any complications that can arise if the infection goes untreated. Along with your doctor's care, here are some things you can do to help yourself.

❖ **Give yourself time to recover.** Rest in bed until the fever and chills stop. Go back to your regular activities when you feel better.

❖ **Use the warm water treatment.** Sit in a shallow tub of warm water for 15 minutes three or more times a day. If you have access to a whirlpool bath, that's even better.

❖ **Exercise your problems away.** Here's an exercise you can do at home to massage your prostate. Lying on your back on a flat surface, place the soles of your feet together with your knees pointing outward. Pull your feet and legs up toward you as far as you can, then return them to the starting position. The movement of your muscles acts as a massage for your prostate gland. Repeat this exercise 10 times in the morning and 10 times at night.

❖ **Stay away from alcohol, tobacco, caffeine, and spicy foods.** These dietary deadbeats can irritate your urethra.

❖ **Drink eight to 10 glasses of water every day.** This will keep your urine flow strong and help prevent kidney infection.

The long-range plan for prostatitis

If you've ever had prostatitis, you know you never want to suffer through it again. Unfortunately, once you've had an infection, the chances are higher that you'll get another one. Here are some steps you can take to keep your prostate healthy enough to fend off the next infection.

❖ **Focus on good nutrition.** Good nutrition can give you the edge against prostatitis. If your body is well-nourished, your immune system can put up a better fight against invading infection.

❖ **Consider vitamin supplements.** Vitamin C and vitamin E play key roles in the health of your prostate gland. Be sure you get at least the recommended daily allowance of these vitamins in the foods you eat, or take a multi-vitamin and mineral supplement if you don't. (See the *Food, vitamin, and mineral chart* on page 351.)

❖ **Zero in on zinc and magnesium.** These two minerals are an important part of your arsenal in the fight against prostatitis. Brewer's yeast, nuts, seeds (especially pumpkin seeds), and wheat germ are good sources of zinc and magnesium.

❖ **Go for the garlic.** Full of vitamins, minerals, and natural antibiotic action, fresh garlic is a delicious and easy-to-use seasoning that promotes prostate health.

❖ **Invest in oil.** Fish oil, contained in fatty fish such as salmon, mackerel, sardines, anchovies, tuna, bluefish, and herring, is a healthy addition to your diet. So are olive oil and evening primrose oil, a natural supplement available at your local health food store. These oils may not only help protect you from prostate problems, but from cancer and heart disease as well.

❖ **Go easy on the needless negatives.** Cut out or cut back on alcohol, tobacco, caffeine, and very spicy foods. These things are irritants, and they counteract some of the helpful effects of vitamins and minerals. Tomatoes and chocolate may irritate your urinary tract as well.

❖ **Drink your water.** Eight to 10 glasses a day are recommended for anyone's good health, but they are especially important when you've had prostate problems.

If prostatitis is the problem causing your sexual pain, you can conquer it and feel good about your sex life again. Research shows that a good way to prevent it is to have an active sex life. So if your wife agrees to frequent lovemaking, you can enjoy yourselves and be protecting your health at the same time — doctor's orders.

⚕ *For women, it's time to see your doctor if you have sexual pain and:*

Tenderness or swelling in your lower abdomen, possibly accompanied by a hard mass that can be felt through your skin

Upset stomach

- Symptoms of anemia (fatigue, paleness, shortness of breath)
- Unexplained weight loss
- Deepening of your voice and excessive growth of body hair

This combination of symptoms could indicate ovarian cancer.

- Feeling ill generally
- Low-grade fever
- Pain in your lower abdomen, on one or both sides
- Bad-smelling discharge from your vagina
- Painful, frequent urination

If you have these symptoms, you may have pelvic inflammatory disease (PID), an infection of your reproductive organs.

- Constant dryness of your mouth, nose, and eyes
- Vaginal dryness that makes intercourse painful
- Painful, achy joints

These symptoms may point to Sjogren's syndrome, an autoimmune disorder. (See also *Mouth dryness* chapter.)

- Genital itching
- Yellowish discharge
- Painful urination

If you have the above symptoms, you may have urethritis, which is an inflammation of your urethra that is usually transmitted sexually.

- Painful, burning, or frequent urination
- Bloody, bad-smelling urine
- Pain in your lower abdomen and lower back
- Low-grade fever

With these symptoms, you may have cystitis, a bladder infection. (See also *Urination, painful* chapter.)

- Pain and itching in and around your vagina
- Painful or burning urination

> Bad-smelling discharge from your vagina

This combination of symptoms probably means you have vaginitis, an inflammation or infection of the vagina. It can be caused by a fungal infection, a tiny parasite, an overgrowth of the bacteria that normally live in the vagina, an allergic reaction, or the thinning and drying of the vaginal lining after menopause.

> A lump in the front or back of your vagina, or sticking out from it
> Uncomfortable urination
> A backache that gets worse when you lift something
> Discomfort in your pelvis
> Difficulty with bowel movements

This could signal a condition called uterine prolapse, which means the muscles holding your uterus have weakened and allowed the uterus to bulge down into your vagina.

The long-range plan for uterine prolapse

If your doctor has diagnosed the cause of your sexual pain as uterine prolapse, don't despair. You were smart to report it to your doctor, and now you can get some help. As many as one in five women past menopause have this condition, but most are too embarrassed to tell their doctors.

The treatment for severe cases is usually a hysterectomy to remove the uterus. However, if you have a milder case, your doctor may prescribe hormone replacement therapy to increase the blood flow to your vaginal tissues and strengthen the tissues that hold your uterus. If you catch uterine prolapse in the early stages, it's much easier to combat, and many of the treatments can be done at home. The same measures work for both treatment and prevention.

❖ **Keep your weight where it should be.** Obesity increases your risk of uterine prolapse. Embark on a healthy weight loss plan if you need to.

303

❖ **Get fit.** Along with maintaining a healthy weight, exercise regularly to keep all your muscles strong. Walking is the perfect exercise if you're out of shape. Just 30 minutes each day, or even three times a week to start, will do wonders for your overall fitness.

❖ **Eat for good health.** Good nutrition affects every part of your body, including your reproductive organs, so be sure you get all the nutrients your body needs. (See the *Food, vitamin, and mineral chart* on page 351.) It's especially important to get lots of fiber in your diet so you can avoid constipation, a condition that aggravates uterine prolapse. Plenty of fresh fruits, fresh vegetables, and whole grain products in your diet should do the trick.

❖ **Kick it with Kegels.** Kegel exercises, also known as pelvic floor exercises, increase the tone of the muscles that hold your uterus in place. To feel the muscles you want to exercise, try stopping your urine stream and then restarting it. These are the muscles you want to use. Once you learn how these muscles feel, contract and relax them for a count of six. Do this several times a day for at least two to three months to get results. This exercise will also help treat and prevent incontinence.

❖ **Put in a pessary.** This device, prescribed by your doctor, is inserted like a diaphragm into your vagina. It can help hold your uterus in place so it doesn't slip farther down.

Over time, the physical strains of childbirth, chronic coughing, and chronic constipation can cause uterine prolapse. So can a job where you do a lot of heavy lifting. But weight problems and lack of exercise are the biggest risk factors. Whatever the cause, catch and treat uterine prolapse as early as you can. Overcoming this problem can improve not only your personal comfort and health, but your sexual enjoyment as well.

Keep the home fires burning

If you have no symptoms other than genital pain, your problem could be a simple one. Dyspareunia is the term for pain during intercourse. If such pain affects one half of a couple, it affects you both, and it may take working together to solve your common problem. Just understanding the situation and some of its causes can go a long way toward finding a solution.

Factors that affect some people as they age can play a part in making sexual intimacy painful. Obesity, joint pain, disease, prescribed medications, and scars from previous surgeries, such as hysterectomies, can all take their toll. You may need to experiment to find the most comfortable sexual positions, even if they're not what you're used to.

If it has been a long time since you've had intercourse, it may be uncomfortable because of physical changes to your body during your abstinence. This is known as the Widow's or Widower's Syndrome. A man may experience impotence and a woman may have vaginal dryness and pain. A patient and cooperative partner can help you reverse this situation. Your doctor or a sex therapist can help, too. Ask for help if you need it.

A woman's sexual pain may be caused by a condition called vaginismus, in which the vaginal muscles contract involuntarily to prevent intercourse. This can result from previous sexual pain, psychological trauma, or a long period of abstinence. Your doctor or sex therapist can give you counseling and muscle retraining exercises to help you relax.

Menopause is a factor that can affect a woman's sexual comfort in a big way. As a woman ages, her vaginal walls become thinner and dryer, and natural lubrication may not be what it once was. If you've gone through "the change," adding a vaginal lubricant may be just what's needed to enhance your comfort and make you feel romantic again. A number of different brands are available today, and some can even be used several hours in advance so you don't have to interrupt the flow of passion.

If you are using a condom, diaphragm, lubricant, or contraceptive foam or gel, one or both of you could be having an allergic reaction to the product. If you have an allergy to lanolin, check for it in the list of ingredients on the label. Try substituting other products to see if an allergy is the problem.

If you don't see any physical reason for your painful intercourse, you may want to look in a different direction. Your brain is the organ that has the greatest influence over your sex life. You can have very real sexual pain without any physical reason.

Depression and lack of self-confidence can chip away at your ability to enjoy sex. So can worry, fatigue, or feelings of anger toward your partner. Spend some time looking at the good things in your life, and get counseling for depression if you think you might need it. Sometimes, just making a list of your problems and blessings can help you get a better perspective.

Spending time with your spouse and doing enjoyable things together are important ways to build your romantic relationship. A happy sex life has as much to do with your life outside the bedroom as inside it. Find ways to appreciate and show love for your spouse, and you may find that romance and comfortable, enjoyable sex are your reward.

Skin problems

Itching
Rash, blisters
Dry, flaky skin
Unexplained sores

Beauty is only skin deep, but if your skin is itchy, red, or blistered, you probably don't feel beautiful or even very happy. If your skin is prone to outbreaks of dryness and itching, take steps to protect it from irritating substances. Wear gloves to protect your hands from detergents and water, use mild soap when bathing, and use a moisturizer every day.

If you have particularly sensitive skin, try wearing only clothes that are made of cotton or cotton blend, since they are less likely to irritate your skin than wool or synthetic fabrics. Though these steps may help, sometimes a skin problem can be more serious than just a little dryness and may require a doctor's attention.

 ## It's time to see the doctor if you have:

- Itching
- Light-red bumps with raised edges that enlarge and spread quickly

You may be suffering from hives, an allergic reaction to food, heat, cold, insect bites, animals, medication, or other substance. Your doctor can determine the cause of the reaction. The hives may disappear within hours or may last much longer. Treat the area with cool compresses, and keep your body as quiet as possible.

- Fever and/or chills
- General ill feeling
- Several days of skin sensitivity or tingling
- Burning or shooting pain
- Blistery, red, itchy rash on the skin most often in a band or strip pattern

These are the symptoms of herpes zoster, more commonly known as shingles. (See also *Face pain* chapter.)

- Redness on the cheeks, nose, chin, or forehead that begins as occasional flare-ups, but gradually becomes more permanent
- Swollen, red, bumpy nose
- Burning, irritated eyes
- Oily skin/pimples
- Dandruff

These symptoms could mean you suffer from rosacea (*rose-AY-see-uh*), a skin disease that is often misdiagnosed as adult acne. (See also *Face rash or flushing* chapter.)

- Patches of thick red skin covered by silvery scales
- Itching (sometimes)
- Arthritis (sometimes)

Scaly patches located mostly on your elbows, knees, scalp, and lower back could indicate psoriasis.

- Round, red, itchy patches

This type of rash is a sign of tinea, or ringworm. It is a kind of fungal infection. If you have tinea on your feet, with cracked, itchy skin between your toes, it is called athlete's foot. If your tinea is in your groin area, it is called jock itch.

The ABCD's of skin cancer

Most skin problems are just annoying or unsightly. However, one problem can be deadly — skin cancer. While most skin cancer is curable if caught early enough, malignant melanoma can be fatal. This form of skin cancer sometimes arises from seemingly innocent moles. To identify this skin disease early enough to cure, learn your ABCD's.

- **A for asymmetry.** This means that one side of a mole doesn't match the other.

- **B for border.** The border of most moles is smooth. A mole with edges that are irregular, ragged, or blurred could be a warning sign.

- **C for color.** A mole that is a mixture of colors, including blue, red, tan, black, white, or brown could be a red flag signalling melanoma.

- **D for diameter.** A mole that is unusually large could also mean cancer. If a mole is larger than a pencil eraser, have it checked out by your doctor.

To protect yourself from skin cancer, the best thing you can do is stay out of the sun and examine your skin regularly. Any change in an existing mole or any new growths should be checked by your doctor.

- Itchiness or pain in the affected area
- Flakiness or blistering
- Redness

This kind of rash could mean you have a form of dermatitis.

Immediate help for dermatitis

Your body has been overtaken by itchy red patches of skin, and you're worried that you look like a kid with chicken pox. However, chances are much greater that you have some form of dermatitis. Dermatitis is the name for several types of skin inflammations.

❖ **Seborrheic dermatitis.** If you avoid wearing black shirts because of embarrassing white flakes on your shoulders, you may have this condition. It is the medical name for what you usually call dandruff in adults or cradle cap in infants. This type of dermatitis makes your skin look greasy and flaky, usually on the scalp. But it can sometimes affect the skin in other areas of your body, like your face or chest. No one is sure what causes seborrheic dermatitis, but it is fairly common and easy to treat with special dandruff shampoos.

❖ **Atopic dermatitis.** This condition is also called atopic eczema. It is a kind of allergic skin condition that tends to be inherited. If other members of your family have the same kind of itching, crusty, thickened areas of skin as you, atopic dermatitis may be the cause. It usually occurs on the face, upper chest, and neck, or on knees, elbows, wrists, and ankles.

❖ **Dermatitis herpetiformis.** Intense itching accompanies patches of tiny red blisters in this chronic disease. It usually develops in adulthood, and may be connected to celiac sprue disease. Celiac sprue involves an allergy to gluten, which is found in many wheat products. Avoiding products that contain gluten may be the key to controlling this type of dermatitis.

❖ **Photodermatitis.** Certain substances can make you more sensitive to sunlight, causing this type of dermatitis. These photosensitizers include certain drugs, perfumes, cosmetics, and plants. If you are sensitive to sunlight, avoid going outside between 10 a.m. and 4 p.m., when the sun is strongest, and always protect your skin with sunscreen.

❖ **Contact dermatitis.** As the name suggests, you have to touch an irritating substance to get this type of dermatitis. You usually don't react immediately, but one to three days afterwards, your skin may become red, itchy, and blistered. A good example is poison ivy. If your skin is sensitive, you may also react to certain metals such as nickel, chrome, and mercury. Other problems include cosmetics, especially permanent hair dyes that contain paraphenylenediamine, and some types of medicated creams or ointments.

The long-range plan for dermatitis

You're a down-to-earth kind of person. You love to work in your yard, and you frequently take long walks in the woods, admiring the plants and the wildlife. However, you have to be careful what kinds of plants you admire. The leaves of a poison ivy plant can leave you with itchy red blisters that make you miserable for days. Poison ivy is the leading cause of contact dermatitis. Its relatives, poison oak and poison sumac, also do their share of making people uncomfortable each year.

Of course, the best way to avoid the annoying itch is to avoid the plants themselves. But to do that, you have to be able to recognize them. "Leaves of three, let it be" is an old saying that warned people away from poison ivy. While this is usually true, sometimes the leaves may grow in groups of five, seven, or even nine, depending on the environment.

Poison ivy has yellow-green flowers and white berries and grows as a vine which may climb up trees, or as a low shrub. Poison oak grows as a small tree or shrub with clusters of yellow berries and leaves that resemble oak leaves. Poison sumac is a rangy shrub that can grow up to 15 feet high. It has seven to 13 smooth-edged leaves and cream-colored berries. It grows mostly in swampy areas.

The sap in these plants has a substance called urushiol that causes the allergic reaction. If the plant is damaged even a little, the urushiol can get on your skin or clothing and set off a reaction. Urushiol can also stick to pets, garden tools, or other objects and then transfer to your skin.

poison ivy

About 85 percent of people will develop an allergic reaction if exposed to the urushiol in poison ivy, oak, and sumac. This allergic sensitivity seems to develop slowly, after being exposed several times, so don't assume that because you've never had a reaction that you are immune. However, you usually become less sensitive as you get older.

To protect yourself before you head for the great outdoors, you might want to try Ivy Block. It's an over-the-counter lotion that protects your skin from poison ivy, poison oak, and poison sumac. Just apply it at least 15 minutes before you go outside.

poison oak

If you know you have been around poison ivy, oak, or sumac, don't waste any time getting it off your skin. You should clean the affected area with rubbing alcohol and rinse with water. Then you should take a shower with soap and warm water. Tools, shoes, or anything else that may have come into contact with the plants should also be wiped with alcohol and rinsed off.

If you don't get your skin cleansed quickly enough, and if you are sensitive to urushiol, redness and swelling will begin in 12 to 48 hours. You will then develop blisters and severe itching, but resist the urge to scratch the blisters if you can. Scratching will not spread your rash, but your fingernails may carry germs which could set off an infection.

poison sumac

After a few days, your rash will become crusty and scaly, and you should be completely healed in 14 to 20 days. In the meantime, if you can't stand the itching, wet compresses or soaking in a cool bath may soothe your itchy skin.

Antihistamine pills may help, and you can buy hydro-cortisone creams over the counter for temporary relief from your itching. If you have a severe reaction, your doctor may prescribe steroid creams or pills.

Slurred speech

The inability to speak clearly

You're having a conversation with a friend, and you notice his speech is a little slurred. Should you be concerned? Yes ... and don't hesitate to seek medical help for your friend. Slurred speech can be an indication of a serious medical problem, especially if it's accompanied by other symptoms.

 ## It's time to see your doctor if you have slurred speech and:

- Muscle weakness or clumsiness
- Fatigue
- Blurred or double vision
- Numbness or tingling
- Incontinence
- Impotence

This combination of symptoms could indicate you have multiple sclerosis, a disorder of the nervous system. It usually begins in early adulthood.

- Paralysis on one side of your face
- Loss of taste on affected side of your face

312

- Earache on affected side of your face
- Numbness on affected side of your face

If you have these symptoms, your slurred speech could be caused by Bell's palsy, a paralysis of your facial muscles that is usually temporary.

- Headache
- Blurred vision or double vision
- Dizziness
- Weakness in your arms or legs

It is possible you may have had a mild stroke, or you may be experiencing a transient ischemic attack (TIA). This temporary brain disturbance usually clears up within 24 hours, but it is a warning sign that something is wrong. See your doctor immediately.

Immediate help for stroke

Don't delay getting help if you have any of the symptoms of a stroke. The sooner you get help, the better your chances of survival without permanent brain damage.

When you have a stroke, the blood supply to your brain is cut off, either by a blockage of blood flow or by a blood vessel that ruptures and bleeds. When the blood supply to your brain is cut off, depriving it of the oxygen it needs, brain cells die.

A stroke that is caused by a blockage is called an ischemic stroke. It is the most common and, fortunately, less deadly type of stroke. Ischemic strokes can be caused by a blood clot that forms in your brain or neck (thrombosis), by a blood clot that forms elsewhere in your body and moves to your brain or neck (embolism), or by a severe narrowing of an artery that won't allow blood through (stenosis).

A stroke that is caused by bleeding into the brain or the area surrounding the brain is called a hemorrhagic stroke. These strokes are more often fatal than ischemic strokes. They are sometimes caused by a ruptured aneurysm — a weakened spot in an artery that bulges outward.

A drug recently approved by the FDA to treat people suffering from strokes makes recovery more likely. This drug, tissue plasminogen activator or tPA (trade name Activase), dissolves blood clots that cause strokes. This will help people who have had an ischemic stroke, but not people who have had a hemorrhagic stroke.

For tPA to be most effective, it must be given within three hours of the stroke. One study found that 12 percent of stroke victims who were given tPA were soon back to normal. These people might otherwise have suffered a lengthy period of disability as a result of their strokes.

Since tPA is a relatively new treatment for stroke, your hospital might not administer it unless you ask for it. It could mean the difference between an independent life and months spent in a wheelchair.

The long-range plan for stroke

Half a million people a year deal with the potentially fatal or crippling effects of stroke. To keep this from happening to you, practice prevention. Don't let a stroke take away your independence or your life.

❖ **Control your blood pressure.** High blood pressure increases your risk of stroke. If you can keep your blood pressure under control, you may avoid a potentially fatal stroke. Your doctor can give you medicine to control your blood pressure, and if you watch your weight, exercise, and limit your salt intake, you should be able to lower the boom on high blood pressure and stroke.

❖ **Chuck the cigarettes.** Smoking contributes to a build-up of fatty substances that can block the main artery that supplies blood to your brain. This type of blockage is the leading cause of strokes in the United States. If that doesn't convince you, consider that the nicotine in cigarettes raises blood pressure, another risk factor for strokes; the carbon monoxide in cigarettes reduces the amount of oxygen that your blood can carry to your brain; and smoking makes your blood thicker and more likely to clot. Kicking the habit isn't easy, but when you consider what smoking is doing to your body, it's worth the effort. Your doctor can recommend programs or medications that may make quitting a little easier.

❖ **Exercise.** Regular exercise can reduce your risk of stroke substantially. Exercise helps to keep your blood pressure under control. One study from Yale University found that men who walked over a mile a day cut their risk of stroke in half.

❖ **Take daily vitamin E and aspirin.** Aspirin has long been recommended for its ability to keep your blood flowing smoothly. Research finds that a daily program of aspirin and vitamin E can reduce your blood's "stickiness" in half. This makes stroke-causing clots less likely to form.

❖ **Keep diabetes under control.** Diabetes can cause damage to blood vessels, making you more likely to become a stroke victim, and if your blood sugar is high when you have a stroke, the resulting brain damage tends to be more severe. If you have diabetes, work to keep your blood sugar under control, and keep your stroke risk at a minimum.

❖ **Don't ignore TIAs.** Transient ischemic attacks are sometimes called mini-strokes. Although the symptoms may only last a short while, they are a warning sign that something is wrong. See your doctor — it could save your life.

Throat soreness

A painful, raw feeling
Intense pain when you swallow

A number of things can give your throat a worked-over feeling — allergies, smoke, alcohol, even sleeping with your mouth open. But if none of these apply, it's probably a virus or bacteria that's causing your problem. The same common virus that gives you a cold can make

315

your throat hurt. And bacteria can bring on throat ailments such as strep.

If you have a viral or bacterial infection, you'll probably have a fever. It's a good rule of thumb to see your doctor if your fever is over 101° F, you have trouble breathing or swallowing, and you have swollen lymph glands in your neck. You should also seek medical help if you have these other combinations of symptoms.

It's time to see your doctor if you have a sore throat and:

- Difficulty swallowing
- Headache
- Fever and chills
- Swollen, tender glands under your jaw or in your neck

These symptoms may indicate you have pharyngitis, an acute inflammation of the throat; or tonsillitis, an acute inflammation of the tonsils. Tonsillitis is usually a childhood disease, but it can also affect adults. Pharyngitis can be the first sign of a more general illness such as flu or mononucleosis.

- Fatigue
- Fever
- An achy, run-down feeling

If you have these symptoms, you may have mononucleosis, a viral infection spread mostly by saliva (which earned it the nickname "kissing disease"). It is especially common among college students.

- Headache
- Cough
- Fever and chills
- Aching muscles
- Fatigue

These symptoms, along with a runny nose, probably mean you have influenza, or "flu," a common respiratory infection. It's caused by a virus and is contagious. (See also *Nose, runny or stuffy* chapter.)

- Difficulty swallowing
- Acid-tasting stomach contents sometimes rise into your mouth when belching
- A burning, heavy, uncomfortable feeling in your chest or upper stomach
- Bloating and gas
- Chronic cough

If you have these symptoms, especially if they get worse at night, you may have gastroesophageal reflux disease (GERD). In this condition, stomach acids back up into your esophagus and irritate the lining, causing an uncomfortable burning sensation. If you suffer from GERD for a long time, your esophagus can suffer severe damage, and it can increase your risk of cancer. Don't just ignore these symptoms. See your doctor. (See also *Heartburn* chapter.)

- Fever
- Swollen, tender glands under your jaw or in your neck
- No symptoms of a cold or flu
- A general ill feeling
- White patches on the back of your throat

If your sore throat developed suddenly, or you were recently exposed to someone with strep throat, you may have strep also. You need to see your doctor for a throat culture.

Immediate help for strep throat

If your illness is diagnosed as strep throat, your doctor will probably prescribe about 10 days' worth of penicillin or other antibiotic to knock out the infection. It's important to follow your doctor's instructions carefully and take your medicine exactly as directed. If you don't, the streptococcus bacteria could come back, and it might cause kidney damage or rheumatic fever, a serious condition that can damage your heart.

Fever — your body's natural fighter

A fever is usually a response to an invading virus or bacteria that multiplies and makes you sick. Its job is to help you fight the infection. If the fever is high, you'll want to bring it down. But if you get rid of it altogether, you'll take away some of your body's natural ability to fight disease.

Here are some tips for dealing with fever:

❖ **Get some rest.** Keep warm, decrease your activity, and sleep if you want to.

❖ **Drink plenty of liquids.** You need at least six to eight cups of liquid a day to prevent dehydration. Try drinking a glass of water or other liquid at least once every hour you're awake.

❖ **Cool down naturally.** Dip a small towel in cool water and wring it out. Use this as a cool compress for the back of your neck or under your arms. Dress lightly and use a sheet as a cover instead of a blanket.

❖ **Pop a pain reliever.** You can use aspirin, ibuprofen, or acetaminophen to relieve your aches and reduce your fever.

❖ **Call your doctor if necessary.** Seek help if you have a temperature over 103° F (or less if you are elderly), a high fever with no sweating, or if your fever lasts more than four days.

Fever can be a real helper and disease fighter. Just be sure to watch it carefully and take it seriously.

Along with your doctor's care, here are some steps you can take to help your body fight off the infection of strep throat.

❖ **If you smoke, stop.** Smoking will irritate your throat even more and might slow your recovery.

❖ **Take it easy.** Bed rest is a good idea if you have a busy, active lifestyle. You need to let your body wrestle with the invading bacteria without having to use so much energy on other physical demands.

❖ **Moisten the air.** Use a cool-mist humidifier in the room you're recuperating in. Moist air can help relieve that parched, scratchy feeling in your throat.

❖ **Drink lots of liquids.** You probably don't feel much like swallowing anything, but liquids are easier on your throat than solids. When you have a fever, you lose a lot of fluid, so it's important to pump plenty of liquids back into your body. You should drink at least six to eight glasses of liquids a day. Drink fruit and vegetable juices, thin soups, herbal and regular teas, and even carbonated drinks and coffee if they appeal to you. But you should emphasize drinks that pack a lot of nutrients rather than empty calories.

❖ **Boost your vitamin C intake.** Some research shows that vitamin C helps fight certain conditions that develop from strep, such as rheumatic fever. People in the tropics, where fruits are rich in vitamin C, rarely get rheumatic fever. Eating fresh fruit or drinking fresh fruit juice is the best way to nourish your body with vitamin C and other antioxidants. (See the *Food, vitamin, and mineral chart* on page 351.)

❖ **Get some garlic.** Because it contains allicin, a natural antibiotic, garlic helps fight the bacteria of strep throat. Fresh garlic works best, so chew two to four cloves when you first notice your sore throat. To tone down garlic breath, you can soak the cloves in yogurt before you eat them, or chew them with a handful of fresh parsley. Fresh onions contain allicin, too, so add a liberal sprinkling to your diet.

❖ **Take some tea.** A strong cup of tea, either warm or cold, makes a soothing gargle for your painful throat. The tannin in tea acts as an astringent on your throat, shrinking blood vessels and swollen tissue. Make your tea twice as strong as you do for drinking, and use it to gargle as often as you like.

❖ **Make a good gargle.** A homemade solution of one-half teaspoon of salt dissolved in a cup of warm water also makes a soothing gargle for your sore throat.

❖ **Try an herbal cure.** Echinacea, an herbal medicine discovered long ago by Native Americans, may have some healing power when it comes to respiratory and strep infections. It also gives your entire immune system a boost. Echinacea is available in drugstores and discount stores in liquid or capsule form.

❖ **Take something for the pain.** Aspirin or ibuprofen can help relieve the pain and inflammation of a strep throat. If you have an ulcer, these pain relievers could upset your stomach, so you might want to rely on the other self-help suggestions instead.

The long-range plan for strep throat

Strep throat is a common illness so it's difficult to avoid, especially if you spend much time around children. You can catch it just from someone breathing or coughing into the air around you. If you know someone has strep throat, it's a good idea to keep your distance and wash your hands often.

The best way to avoid getting a case of strep throat is to keep your immune system strong. Then, when you're exposed to the streptococcus bacteria, your body's own defenses can fend it off. Eating nutritious foods, getting enough sleep, and exercising regularly will give your body's immune system its best fighting chance.

If you have the symptoms of strep throat, don't put off medical care or try to be tough. Go to your doctor and have a strep test. He can easily find out whether your throat pain is due to a strep throat or something that will simply run its course and fade away on its own. Either way, your sore throat should soon be nothing more than a distant memory.

Trembling

Uncontrollable shaking

You're all shook up, trembling uncontrollably, and you want an explanation. It could be from the cold, from fright, or simply from too much caffeine. However, sometimes trembling doesn't have such simple explanations, and you need to see your doctor for answers.

 ## It's time to see your doctor if you have trembling and:

- Weakness and fatigue
- Unexplained weight loss
- Bulging eyes
- Are overly active
- Feel generally warm or hot

You may be suffering from hyperthyroidism, also called thyrotoxicosis, toxic goiter, or Graves' disease. This is a relatively common disorder caused by an overactive thyroid. (See also **Weight changes, unexplained** chapter.)

- Nausea or vomiting (especially in the morning)
- Memory problems, confusion
- Red face
- Personality changes
- Frequent intoxication

The above symptoms may be a warning signal that you have a problem with alcohol dependence.

- Brief, recurrent periods of severe facial pain
- Red face
- Teary eye

You may have trigeminal neuralgia. Because the severe pain causes facial wincing, this condition is

321

commonly called tic douloureux, meaning "painful twitch."

- Stiffness
- Slowness of movement
- Speech problems
- Fatigue
- Depression

These symptoms could mean you have Parkinson's disease.

Immediate help for Parkinson's disease

What did Harry Truman and Adolf Hitler have in common? Besides having a profound effect on history, both these men had Parkinson's disease.

Parkinson's mainly affects people over the age of 40, but it can occasionally strike younger people. It is a disorder in which your brain cells, or neurons, break down. These neurons produce a chemical that helps your brain control your muscle movements. When they die, they no longer make the chemical, called dopamine, and your muscles don't work as well.

The early symptoms of Parkinson's disease are general and easy to overlook. At first you may simply feel tired and weak. Then you may notice that your hands tremble while at rest. This is one of the most common symptoms of Parkinson's. Your muscles may begin to feel stiff, you may move more slowly, and you may have trouble keeping your balance. You might notice a change in your speech, or your handwriting may become much smaller.

If you think you may have Parkinson's, see your doctor. He can prescribe medicine that will help you. The most common is Levodopa, or L-dopa, which changes to dopamine in your brain. However, L-dopa becomes less effective the longer you use it, so you should try to delay taking this medication as long as possible.

The long-range plan for Parkinson's disease

A diagnosis of Parkinson's disease is not the end of the line. Treatments are available, researchers continue to search for a cure, and you have the ability to take control of this disease.

❖ **Exercise.** If you've always been a physically active person, you're a step ahead of the game. If you haven't been active, it's not too late to start. The earlier in your disease you begin an exercise program, the better. You may be able to delay some of the stiffness and fatigue that Parkinson's causes. Aerobic and strengthening exercises are both beneficial, but just taking a walk every day can help. Ask your doctor or physical therapist to recommend an appropriate exercise program.

❖ **Watch what you eat.** Some people with Parkinson's find that certain foods make their symptoms worse. For example, hot, spicy foods may make movement more difficult. Keep track of what you eat, and note whether it seems to have any effect on your symptoms.

Research finds that protein can interfere with your body's absorption of L-dopa. If you are taking L-dopa, you may want to eat less protein,

Surgery for Parkinson's

You may have heard that surgery is now available for Parkinson's disease. Before you rush out to find a neurosurgeon, however, make sure you get all the facts.

"Pallidotomy" involves cutting a small hole in your skull and destroying a select group of cells deep within your brain. This surgery is not for you if medication is controlling your symptoms. It is recommended for people who responded well to medication at first but had problems with it later on. Surgery also is not recommended for people who have memory loss, confusion, or disorientation.

Pallidotomy often improves many of the symptoms of Parkinson's and helps many people remain active longer. But it is not a cure. Most people still need their anti-Parkinson medication following surgery.

but don't eat too little. You may become deficient. Try eating smaller amounts of protein with carbohydrates several times during the day. Or eat most of your protein at night when your medicine doesn't have to be as effective. Broad beans, also known as fava beans, may be one protein source that doesn't interfere with your L-dopa as much.

Constipation can be a side effect of Parkinson's, so make sure you get plenty of fiber, and drink lots of water. Talk to your doctor about your eating plan, and experiment until you find what works best for you.

❖ **Get some support.** You may have a caring family, but they cannot quite understand what you're going through. Other people with Parkinson's do understand. Joining a support group may help keep you from feeling alone and depressed, and you may get some helpful advice on how other people have dealt with the disease.

❖ **Think about therapy.** Different types of therapy are available to people with Parkinson's. Physical therapy may help teach you how to deal with your movement problems and increase your mobility. Some people with Parkinson's have speech difficulties because the muscles in your throat and voice box don't work properly. Speech therapy may help you speak more clearly, and make your disease less noticeable. Psychological counseling may help you overcome the depression that so often accompanies Parkinson's.

❖ **Gadgets can be helpful.** Handy little gadgets like jar openers, reachers, and special cooking and eating utensils can make your life much easier, and help you to stay independent.

❖ **Make your home safe.** Because Parkinson's can affect your balance, it is important to fall-proof your home. Install hand rails and non-skid strips in your bathroom, because a fall in the bathtub can be disastrous. Keep your floors free of clutter that might trip you up, and have night lights throughout your house, especially along the path you would take to the bathroom at night.

For more help dealing with Parkinson's disease, call the American Parkinson Disease Association at 1-800-223-2732, or write them at 60 Bay Street, Staten Island, NY, 10301. They have a number of pamphlets with lots of useful information for people with Parkinson's.

Urination, frequent

Urinating more than four to six times daily
Awakening several times at night to urinate

If you've worn a path in the carpet between your bedroom and your bathroom, or if you can't go on a car trip without stopping at every gas station along the way to use the facilities, you may have a problem with frequent urination. While it may not sound like a serious problem, frequent urination can be a warning signal that you shouldn't ignore.

 ## It's time to see your doctor if you have frequent urination and:

- Excessive thirst
- Increased appetite
- Unexplained weight loss
- Frequent infections
- Fatigue

If you have these symptoms, you may have diabetes. (See also *Weight changes, unexplained* chapter.)

- Painful, burning urination
- Bloody, bad-smelling urine
- Pain in your lower abdomen and lower back
- Low-grade fever

325

With these symptoms, you may have a bladder infection or other urinary tract infection. (See also *Urination, painful* chapter.)

For women:
- Feel ill generally
- Low-grade fever
- Pain in your lower abdomen, on one or both sides
- Bad-smelling discharge from your vagina
- Painful urination

These are symptoms of pelvic inflammatory disease (PID), an infection of your reproductive organs.

For men:
- Problems in beginning the urine stream and emptying your bladder
- Fever and chills
- Low back pain
- Achy muscles and joints
- Unusual discharge from your penis

These symptoms could point to an infection of your prostate gland, known as prostatitis; a sexually transmitted disease, such as gonorrhea; or an infection of your urethra, the tube that carries urine from your bladder. (See also *Sexual pain* chapter.)

- Problems in beginning the urine stream
- Weak urine stream
- Feel as if your bladder is never completely emptied
- "Dribbling" after urination

These symptoms may indicate that you have benign prostatic hyperplasia (BPH), which is an enlarged prostate, or prostate cancer.

Immediate help for prostate disease

Benign prostatic hyperplasia (BPH) is extremely common in older men. It affects about half the men over age 60 and 90 percent of men who are 85 years old. BPH can cause serious urinary problems because it can interfere with the flow of urine. Having BPH does not make you more likely to get prostate cancer, although you can have both conditions.

Your prostate surrounds your urethra at the point where it leaves the bladder. Your urethra's job is to carry urine and semen out of your body. Your prostate's main job is to contribute fluid to the semen.

When your prostate develops hyperplasia, which means it has too many cells and is enlarged, it can put the squeeze on your urethra, making urination more difficult. This can cause your urine to back up into your bladder, making infection more likely. The increased pressure on your kidneys or the spread of infection from your bladder to your kidneys can cause kidney damage. You may also develop painful bladder stones.

Occasionally, men with BPH find they are suddenly unable to urinate at all. This is called acute urinary retention, and it requires immediate medical attention. Your doctor will insert a catheter to drain the urine from your bladder.

Treatment options for BPH include watchful waiting, medication, and surgery. If your BPH is only causing you some inconvenience because of your frequent trips to the bathroom, you may decide to opt for watchful waiting. This simply means doing nothing while keeping a close eye on your prostate by having regular checkups with your doctor.

Medicine for the treatment of BPH hasn't been around long, so the long-term effects are still being studied. Early research finds that prostate drugs improve symptoms in about 30 to 60 percent of the men who take them. Finasteride, the most common drug used to treat BPH, seems to be effective and has few side effects. Of the men who take it, 3 to 4 percent may experience impotence.

When BPH is causing serious urinary problems, your doctor may encourage you to have your prostate surgically removed, called prostatectomy. A prostatectomy for BPH usually removes only the inner tissue of the prostate (simple prostatectomy), while one done for prostate cancer removes the entire organ (radical prostatectomy).

Surgery usually offers the best chance for relief from urinary symptoms, but it may not be a cure-all. A prostatectomy will not correct bladder damage suffered as a result of your BPH, so you may continue to have symptoms. Surgery also can cause long-term side effects, including impotence, incontinence, and retrograde ejaculation. This is when your semen ejaculates back into your bladder instead of out your penis. A second operation is required in about 10 percent of the men who have prostatectomies.

The future may be brighter. Recent advances in surgical procedures might reduce the chances of these side effects.

The long-range plan for prostate disease

BPH isn't the only disease that affects your prostate. Prostate cancer is also common among older men. According to one estimate, about 60 to 70 percent of the men who live to the age of 80 have some degree of prostate cancer. Since people are living longer than ever before, the cases of prostate cancer are expected to rise as more men reach their 70s and 80s. If you live into your 80s, you need a long-range plan for avoiding prostate cancer. While you can't do much about the main risk factors for prostate cancer, age and family history, there are still some things you can do to help lower your risk of this dreaded disease.

❖ **Watch the fat.** According to Harvard researchers, the more high-fat foods men eat, the more likely they are to have prostate tumors that advance to the life-threatening stage. This was especially true for men who ate a lot of red meat. These men were two-and-a-half times as likely to develop advanced tumors.

❖ **Soak up some rays.** Early research indicates that exposure to sunlight may help protect against prostate cancer by helping your body produce vitamin D. One study found that deaths from prostate cancer were highest where exposure to sunlight was lowest. Get at least a half hour of sunlight every day if you can. It's the best way to ensure that your body will produce vitamin D. It is difficult to get enough vitamin D from food, and supplements can be toxic if you take too much. If you do take supplements, the recommended amount is 400 to 800 International Units (IU) daily.

❖ **Eat more tomatoes.** Researchers find that tomato-based products like tomato sauce and pizza may help protect your prostate. A Harvard study found that men who ate at least 10 servings of tomato-based products a week reduced their risks of prostate cancer by 45 percent. Lycopene, the substance that gives tomatoes their red color, is probably responsible for this protective effect.

❖ **See your doctor regularly.** As with most cancers, prostate cancer is easier to cure in the early stages. If it spreads, your chances of survival drop sharply. Your doctor may be able to feel a tumor during a digital rectal exam (DRE). He may also give you a prostate specific antigen (PSA) test. PSA is an enzyme that is secreted into your prostatic ducts during ejaculation. Normally, very little PSA enters your bloodstream. If you have an abnormality in your prostate, like a tumor, more of the enzyme may escape into your bloodstream. A PSA test cannot tell for sure whether you have prostate cancer. While BPH and prostatitis can cause your PSA level to rise, some men with prostate cancer don't have elevated PSA levels. A PSA of 4 ng/ml (nanograms per milliliter of blood) is generally considered normal. If you have a PSA between 4 and 10 ng/ml, the chance that you have prostate cancer is 20 to 50 percent. If your PSA level is over 10 ng/ml, you are 50 to 75 percent more likely to have prostate cancer, and if your PSA level goes over 20, there is a 90 percent chance that you have prostate cancer. Although the PSA test is not foolproof, it is one of the best tools your doctor has for detecting a tumor in your prostate before it has a chance to spread. New testing techniques are helping to make the PSA test more reliable. For example, researchers have discovered that ejaculation causes your PSA level to rise temporarily, which could cause a false reading. Doctors now recommend that you abstain from sex for at least two days before getting a PSA test.

Urination, painful

A burning or stinging pain when you urinate

It's a routine part of every day. You usually don't give it a second thought — until it becomes painful. If you dread going to the bathroom, and sometimes put off going as long as possible just to avoid the pain, burning, and stinging, you need to find out what's wrong.

 It's time to see your doctor if you have painful urination and:

For men:
- Problems in beginning the urine stream and emptying your bladder
- Fever and chills
- Low back pain
- Achy muscles and joints
- Unusual discharge from your penis

These symptoms could point to an infection of your prostate gland, known as prostatitis; a sexually transmitted disease, such as gonorrhea; or an infection of your urethra, the tube that carries urine from your bladder. (See also *Sexual pain* chapter.)

For women:
- Feel ill generally
- Low-grade fever
- Pain in your lower abdomen, on one or both sides

330

- Bad-smelling discharge from your vagina
- Painful intercourse

If you have these symptoms, you may have pelvic inflammatory disease (PID), an infection of your reproductive organs.

- A lump in the front or back of your vagina, or sticking out from it
- A backache that gets worse when you lift something
- Discomfort in your pelvis
- Difficulty with bowel movements

This could indicate a condition called uterine prolapse, which means the muscles holding your uterus have weakened and allowed the uterus to bulge down into your vagina. (See also *Sexual pain* chapter.)

- Pain and itching in and around your vagina
- Painful sexual intercourse
- Bad-smelling discharge from your vagina

This combination of symptoms probably means you have vaginitis, an inflammation or infection of the vagina. It can be caused by a fungal infection, a tiny parasite, an overgrowth of the bacteria that normally live in the vagina, an allergic reaction, or the thinning and drying of the vaginal lining after menopause.

For both sexes:
- Painful intercourse
- Blisters or sores on the skin of your genital area
- Swollen lymph glands in your groin

This may indicate an infection or inflammation of your skin, such as genital herpes, which is a viral infection.

- You have had a strong blow to your lower abdomen
- Blood in your urine or inability to urinate

331

- Pain in lower abdomen

These symptoms indicate that the blow to your abdomen may have injured your bladder.

- Genital itching
- Yellowish discharge
- Painful intercourse

If you have these symptoms, you may have urethritis, which is an inflammation of your urethra. The disease is usually transmitted sexually.

- Frequent urination
- Bloody, bad-smelling urine
- Pain in your lower abdomen and lower back
- Low-grade fever

With these symptoms, you may have a bladder infection or a kidney infection.

Immediate help for urinary tract infections

How would you feel if your body was invaded by foreign substances intent on causing harm? That's exactly what happens when you get an infection. Tiny disease-causing microorganisms, like bacteria or viruses, enter your body and begin to multiply. Your body has its own army of cells that attack foreign invaders, but sometimes it needs extra ammunition. A particularly common type of infection your body may need help fighting off is a urinary tract infection (UTI).

Your urinary tract includes your kidneys, ureters, bladder, and urethra. Your kidneys' main job is to filter your blood, pulling out liquid waste in the form of urine. Your kidneys also keep the acid levels in your body balanced, and they produce several important hormones. Your ureters are tubes that take urine from your kidneys to your bladder, where it is stored until you urinate. At that time, the urine moves down your urethra and out of your body.

Although urine is normally sterile — it has no bacteria, viruses, or fungi — bacteria still manage to get into your urinary tract.

Most urinary tract infections begin in the urethra since it is closest to outside sources of bacteria. UTIs are much more common in women, probably because they have a much shorter urethra than men, and their urethra is located close to their anus and vagina, which are both potential sources of bacteria.

Any type of blockage in the urinary system may result in an infection. If urine cannot be emptied out of your body quickly, it may stagnate, giving bacteria an opportunity to grow. In men, a common cause of this is an enlarged prostate gland that restricts the flow of urine. Bladder stones sometimes form in your bladder and may set off an infection. A bladder tumor can have the same effect.

If you're a woman, not only are you more likely to have a UTI, you are also more likely to have repeated UTIs. Of the women who get a UTI, 20 percent will have another one, and if you've already had three UTIs, your chances of having yet another one is 80 percent.

If you have the symptoms of a UTI, don't just assume it will clear up on its own. Bladder infections usually only cause temporary discomfort, but if the infection spreads to your kidneys, it can cause permanent kidney damage or result in blood poisoning, which can be fatal.

It's important that you see your doctor. If his diagnosis is a UTI, he will probably prescribe an antibiotic to help your body fight off the infection.

The long-range plan for urinary tract infections

If you're familiar with the pain of a urinary tract infection, chances are you've taken your fair share of antibiotics. Antibiotics are effective weapons against infections, but only if you take all of them. If you don't finish taking your antibiotics, you may have only injured the bacteria. They might regroup in a slightly different form and attack again.

Doctors are becoming very concerned that antibiotics are not the potent weapon against infection they once were. You can help yourself and others by always finishing your antibiotics, and trying to avoid getting an infection in the first place by following these suggestions.

- ❖ **Drink plenty of water.** Drinking lots of water may help wash bacteria from your urinary tract.
- ❖ **Chug some cranberry juice.** Drinking cranberry juice is an old home remedy for UTIs, but many doctors think it really helps. If you drink enough of it, cranberry juice makes your urine more acidic, which makes it more difficult for bacteria to grow.
- ❖ **Add some C.** Vitamin C may also help acidify your urine, so if you can't stand cranberry juice, taking vitamin C supplements might help.
- ❖ **Go whenever you feel the need.** You may be tempted to resist the urge to urinate if you think it's going to be painful, or even if you're just too busy to bother. Just remember, the longer urine sits in your bladder, the more time bacteria have to multiply.
- ❖ **Wipe carefully.** Women should take special care to wipe from front to back. If you wipe from back to front, you may drag bacteria from your anus forward to your urethra, giving germs easy access to set off an infection.
- ❖ **Ditch the tub.** Tub baths may be relaxing, but sitting in the water may give bacteria an opportunity to enter your body. Take showers instead whenever possible.
- ❖ **Keep it clean.** Wash your genital area before having sexual intercourse. This may help prevent spreading bacteria from one person to the other.
- ❖ **Choose birth control carefully.** Studies find that women who use diaphragms for birth control are more likely to get urinary tract infections. Recent evidence also indicates that women whose partners use condoms with spermicidal foam may also have a higher risk of infection.
- ❖ **Go unscented.** Scented douches and feminine hygiene sprays may smell pretty, but they may also irritate your urethra.
- ❖ **Avoid irritants.** Certain foods and beverages may irritate your bladder. Common offenders include

coffee, tea, alcohol, carbonated beverages, and spicy foods.

❖ **Stop smoking.** In case you need another good reason to get rid of your cigarettes, the leading cause of bladder cancer is smoking.

Weight changes, unexplained

Loss of weight without dieting or exercising
Weight gain with no changes in diet or exercise habits

Most people have to struggle to keep their weight down. However, sometimes gaining weight means something other than too many twinkies in front of the TV. For example, many prescription drugs, including birth control pills, can cause weight gain as a side effect. Hormonal changes like the ones experienced in menopause can often result in bloating and weight gain.

While weight loss may be a more desirable alternative for most people, unexplained weight loss can also mean something is wrong. You may yearn to lose a lot of weight without dieting or exercise, but if it actually happens you should probably be concerned. Unexplained weight loss can result from diseases as serious and deadly as AIDs and cancer. If you suddenly start dropping pounds for no apparent reason, don't go out and celebrate until you've seen your doctor.

⚕ It's time to see your doctor if you have:

- Loss of appetite, weight loss
- Anxiety, mood swings

- Lack of enjoyment in activities or life in general
- Difficulty sleeping
- Thoughts of death or suicide
- Feelings of sadness or hopelessness

Depression is a common condition, especially as you age. Physical problems such as an illness, medication, or hormonal changes, can bring it on. So can social or psychological factors. Don't feel you have to fight it alone. Get help as soon as possible. (See also *Depression* chapter.)

- Unexplained weight loss
- Abdominal pain spasms
- Fever

If your battles with diarrhea seem to come and go, and you also have the above symptoms, you may have Crohn's disease. No one knows what causes this chronic disease, but the number of people affected by it seem to be increasing.

- Excessive weight loss
- Nausea and vomiting
- Gas and bloating
- Rectal itching

If you have these symptoms, you may have an intestinal parasite. The thought of worms may be unpleasant, but it can happen to the best of us.

- Unexplained weight loss
- Fatigue
- Vomiting
- Abdominal pain

These are the symptoms of a rare disorder called celiac sprue disease. This disease causes gluten to damage the lining of your small intestine. Gluten is a protein found in wheat, barley, and rye, and the only treatment is to avoid all foods that have it. Rice, corn, and soybean flour are good substitutes. The only way to diagnose the disease is to see your doctor.

336

- Loss of appetite (which may lead to weight loss)
- Cramping abdominal pain that is usually relieved by bowel movements
- Diarrhea alternating with constipation
- Nausea

These symptoms may mean you have irritable bowel syndrome (IBS). IBS is usually just an annoyance and does not cause any serious damage. But if it interferes with your lifestyle by keeping you away from public functions, discuss it with your doctor. (See also *Diarrhea* chapter.)

- Unexplained weight loss
- Weakness and fatigue
- Hyperactivity
- Rapid, irregular heartbeat
- Increased sweating
- Bulging eyes

You may be suffering from hyperthyroidism, also called thyrotoxicosis, toxic goiter, or Graves' disease. This is a relatively common disorder caused by an overactive thyroid. It can usually be controlled by medication.

- Weight gain or extreme thinness
- Decreased appetite, sweating, and tolerance for cold
- Chest pain
- Sleepiness or insomnia
- Mental problems like depression or poor memory

These symptoms might indicate hypothyroidism, an underactive thyroid. Although hypothyroidism is generally easy to treat with thyroid replacement drugs, it can cause life-threatening complications in rare cases, so it is important to see your doctor.

- Unexplained weight loss
- Increased appetite
- Excessive thirst
- Frequent urination
- Fatigue

⁘ Frequent infections

These symptoms may mean you have diabetes.

Immediate help for diabetes

You've been overweight most of your life. You've tried every fad diet that comes along but just can't seem to keep the pounds off. Suddenly, however, you're miraculously dropping pounds with no effort. But you're not sleeping well because you're constantly popping up for a glass of water or a trip to the bathroom. Your next trip should be to your doctor's office, because you have several symptoms of diabetes.

There are two types of diabetes, Type I insulin-dependent diabetes mellitus (IDDM), and Type II non-insulin-dependent diabetes mellitus (NIDDM). Type I diabetes occurs when your pancreas doesn't make enough insulin or stops making insulin altogether. If you don't have enough insulin to keep your blood sugar under control, you will die, so daily insulin shots are necessary. Type II diabetes is less serious and far more common. It develops more slowly and can usually be controlled through diet and lifestyle changes, but sometimes medication is necessary.

If your doctor confirms the diagnosis, take comfort in the fact that you are not alone. Approximately 16 million people in the United States have diabetes. About half of them do not realize they have the condition.

Although many diabetics today lead happy, normal lives, it is still a serious disorder. It contributes to the deaths of almost 200,000 people a year and is the leading cause of new blindness among adults. If you think you have diabetes, the best thing you can do is get tested by your doctor. Then you can take steps to protect yourself from the potentially devastating effects of this disease.

The long-range plan for diabetes

Nine out of ten people who get diabetes will have Type II non-insulin-dependent diabetes. Fortunately, this type is easier to control and usually not as dangerous as Type I diabetes. Although heredity may play a part in who gets Type II diabetes, it is usually brought on by another factor such as obesity. Therefore, you have some control over whether you get the disease and how seriously it will affect you.

Check out your thyroid

If you have gained or lost weight unexpectedly, a small butterfly-shaped gland near the base of your neck could be responsible. Your thyroid gland produces hormones that regulate your metabolism. If it makes too much of these hormones, your metabolism speeds up and you have hyperthyroidism. If it doesn't produce enough, your metabolism slows down and causes hypothyroidism. The only way to tell for sure is to have your doctor test your thyroid.

Hyperthyroidism. If your thyroid is overactive, you may feel jittery and anxious, "wired" but tired. You may notice that your hands tremble, that you sweat a lot and can't stand the heat. You may have occasional heart palpitations, sleep disturbances, vision problems, and more frequent bowel movements.

Hyperthyroidism increases your risk of heart disease and osteoporosis, and it can cause vision problems. It can be treated with drugs, by a radioactive iodine drink that destroys part of your thyroid, or by surgically removing part of your thyroid.

Hypothyroidism. If your thyroid is sluggish, you may feel drained and depressed, forgetful, and unable to concentrate. Your skin may be dry, yellowish, and cold. Your voice may be hoarse, and you could begin to lose your hair.

Luckily, hypothyroidism is fairly easy to control with synthetic hormones. The American Association of Clinical Endocrinologists recommends that women over 40 (who are most likely to have hypothyroidism) be routinely screened for thyroid problems.

❖ **Keep your weight down.** You are most at risk for developing Type II diabetes if you are over the age of 40, have a family history of diabetes, and are overweight. You can't help the first two, but you can control your weight. Although maintaining a healthy weight is important for everyone, it may be especially important if diabetes runs in your family.

❖ **Eat more salmon.** A little pink fish on your plate could save you from diabetes. One study found that people who ate salmon every day were 50 percent less likely to get diabetes as people who didn't eat salmon.

❖ **Exercise.** If you have diabetes, you can benefit from regular exercise in several ways. It helps you maintain a healthy weight and it can lower your blood sugar level. Exercise can also reduce your risk of heart disease, which is important since diabetics have a much higher risk of heart disease than most people. Always consult your doctor before you begin an exercise program.

❖ **Stick to your food plan.** Your doctor or dietician will work with you to develop a food plan. Diabetics were once required to follow a strict diet with very little sugar. However, The American Diabetes Association issued new guidelines for diabetic eating plans in 1994. These guidelines reflected new knowledge about diabetes and nutrition. You can now enjoy an occasional sweet as long as you adjust the rest of your diet accordingly. But don't let tempting goodies wreck your food plan and destroy your health.

❖ **Eat smaller, more frequent meals.** According to a recent study, diabetics who ate four to six small meals instead of three large ones lowered their blood sugar levels and required less insulin.

❖ **Get plenty of fiber.** A high-fiber diet can help you regulate your blood sugar. When increasing your fiber intake, make sure you drink at least six glasses of water daily to prevent constipation.

❖ **Give up the cigarettes and alcohol.** Smoking damages your pancreas, which you need to produce insulin. Alcohol can cause hypoglycemia (low blood sugar) and interact with your medicine.

❖ **Take some vitamin C.** A humble vitamin may help prevent the damaging effects of diabetes. A recent study found that diabetics who took 500 milligrams (mg) of vitamin C twice a day lowered their cholesterol levels as well as their levels of cell-damaging free radicals. Another study found that 1,000 mg of daily vitamin C strengthened blood vessels in the hands, feet, kidneys, and retinas of people with diabetes. Since most diabetes complications involve damaged blood vessels, vitamin C could help protect you from some serious side effects.

Wheezing

Tightness in your chest and breathing difficulty
A whistling sound from your lungs when you breathe

It would almost be funny if it weren't so frightening — that weird, whistling sound your breathing makes when you suddenly begin to wheeze. You hear it from young children along with the strange, barking cough of croup. Asthmatics make the sound when they suffer an attack. Whatever the cause of your wheezing, it's a symptom you shouldn't ignore.

 ## It's time to see your doctor if you have wheezing and:

Sudden swelling of your face, hands, mouth, or throat
Itching all over
Coughing or sneezing

- Faintness or weakness
- Pounding or rapid heartbeat
- Numbness or tingling around your mouth

These symptoms indicate anaphylaxis, a severe allergic reaction. They can occur within a few seconds to a few minutes after you're exposed to a substance you're allergic to. This is a medical emergency; loss of consciousness may be the next symptom to occur. If you have these symptoms, get medical help immediately.

- Rapid breathing and shortness of breath
- Sweating and paleness
- Cough with white, brown, or frothy pink sputum
- Leg swelling

If you wake up in the night with these symptoms, you may have pulmonary edema, or fluid in your lungs. This is a life-threatening condition associated with congestive heart failure. Get medical help immediately.

- Coughing
- Chest pain
- Unexplained weight loss
- Weakness and fatigue

Together, these symptoms could indicate lung cancer.

- Persistent cough
- Burning or pressure in your chest
- Thick sputum that is difficult to cough up

These symptoms, especially a persistent cough and difficult breathing, could mean your lungs or bronchial tubes are inflamed. If you work in a dusty place, you might have asbestosis, silicosis, or pneumoconiosis. In a dust-free environment, it could be bronchiectasis or chronic bronchitis. Bronchitis can attack year after year or become a permanent health problem known as chronic obstructive pulmonary disease (COPD). (See also *Coughing* chapter.)

- Coughing
- Low-grade fever
- Burning or pressure in your chest

If you have a cough that won't let up, which starts out dry then includes gray or yellow sputum, you may have acute bronchitis, an inflammation of the air passages of the lungs. (See also *Coughing* chapter.)

- Tightness in your chest
- Shortness of breath
- A dry cough, especially at night

The frequent recurrence of these symptoms, along with wheezing, may indicate that you have bronchial asthma.

Immediate help for asthma

Bronchial asthma is a chronic condition that causes attacks of breathlessness and wheezing. Your bronchial tubes swell up and lung secretions increase, which temporarily lessens or closes off the air to your lungs.

If you have asthma, you may be allergic to substances outside your body (extrinsic or allergic asthma). Or some unknown factor within your body can cause it (intrinsic or chronic asthma). Although it's usually thought of as a childhood disease, it can develop at any time in your life. As many as 15 percent of people in the United States over the age of 45 have some form of asthma.

Once your doctor has diagnosed your condition, you need to follow the health care plan she has set out for you. The actions you take and the way you manage your environment can have a huge impact on your asthma and how comfortable it is to live with. Try our tips and techniques to give asthma a bit part rather than a starring role in your life.

- ❖ **Watch for the warning signs.** When you feel tired and get a headache, itchy throat, runny nose, and a funny feeling in your chest, chances are you're about to have an asthma attack. Other common warning signals are breathing changes, feeling easily upset, glassy eyes, dark circles under your eyes, paleness, sweating, coughing, sneezing, and dry mouth. Whatever your specific signals, get familiar with them so you'll have some advance notice when an attack is coming.

❖ **Have a plan of attack.** Keep your asthma medicine with you at all times so you're prepared for an attack. During an asthma attack, sit upright. This helps you breath a little easier than when you're lying down. If the attack comes on after you've been exercising, rest and sip some warm water to help thin secretions. Use your bronchodilator as your doctor has recommended.

❖ **Know the difference between an attack and a medical emergency.** You may be accustomed to asthma attacks and know exactly how to deal with them. But a really severe attack can be life-threatening. Watch out for these symptoms:

● You cough or wheeze continuously.

● You have severe shortness of breath or tight-ness in your chest.

● Your breathing slows or becomes shallow and fast.

● Your shoulders hunch over as you try to catch your breath.

● Your nostrils flare as you breathe.

● It becomes difficult to talk or concentrate.

● The skin around your mouth looks slightly gray or blue.

These are signs of a serious asthma attack. You need to get medical treatment immediately. Make plans with your family ahead of time so they'll know how to get help quickly if such an emergency should arise.

The long-range plan for asthma

Managing your asthma on a day-to-day basis takes time and effort, but it will give you more control of your life. It's important to identify triggers in your environment so you can avoid them as much as possible. These are the things that cause your asthma to flare up. Here are some steps you can take to minimize the impact asthma has on your life.

❖ **Prepare for the season.** If you have asthma, plan your most important events for summer. It's probably the best and healthiest season for you. In a study based on hospital admissions for asthma, researchers found September and October were the worst months for asthma patients. Springtime can also cause problems. Knowing this, you can try to avoid triggers and take better care of yourself during the riskiest times of the year.

❖ **Watch the weather.** Changing weather conditions can affect your asthma. Strong winds and changes in temperature, humidity, and barometric pressure may help trigger an asthma attack. So can weather inversions that trap pollution and ozone near the ground. Thunderstorms can be a trigger, too. In 1994, more than 600 people in England were plunged into an asthma epidemic when a high grass pollen count and a huge thunderstorm combined to trigger asthma, even in some people who never had it before. Watch out for high pollen or pollution counts in your area, and stay inside when the numbers are large.

❖ **Avoid chemical irritants.** Household products such as bleach, furniture polish, paints, and perfumes can trigger an asthma attack. Cooking fumes, especially from frying, and dusty substances such as talcum powder and chalk can irritate, too. Try to get someone else in your household to deal with these products, or try to find less-irritating substitutes.

❖ **Sniff out sulfites.** For people with asthma, sulfites, used to preserve food and sanitize drink containers, can cause a real problem. Commonly found in many supermarket foods, sulfites can trigger a severe asthma attack in someone who is sensitive to them. They can also cause symptoms such as hives, itching, flushing, tingling, and nausea. By order of the Food and Drug Administration, you can now tell whether packaged food contains sulfites by reading the list of ingredients. Watch out

Anaphylaxis — when allergy turns deadly

If you have a severe allergy to peanuts, you may want to think twice about traveling by airplane. A recent study showed that air filters in planes may contain enough airborne particles of peanuts to cause a serious reaction in an allergic person. Although this allergic reaction, known as anaphylaxis, is rare, it is sometimes fatal.

Shellfish, peanuts, eggs, milk, celery, legumes (peas and beans), and food additives such as sulfites can cause anaphylaxis in people who are sensitive to them. Drugs, especially penicillin, muscle relaxants, and seizure medications, are a leading cause of anaphylactic shock.

Latex (as in surgical gloves), blood transfusions, and some fluids given after surgery can also set off this reaction. A bee, hornet, yellow jacket, or wasp sting, which quickly injects an allergic substance into your body, can be harmful as well.

So how can you protect yourself? If you've ever had anaphylaxis, you should carry an emergency injection of epinephrine with you at all times. This little kit, called Ana-Kit or EpiPen, is available by prescription from your doctor. If you do use an injection to prevent anaphylaxis, go to an emergency room immediately afterward. The epinephrine only lasts for about an hour. When it wears off, your symptoms may return.

You can also wear a Medic Alert bracelet, which carries a warning to inform rescuers about your allergy even if you're unconscious. For information, write to: Medic Alert, P.O. Box 1009, Turlock, CA 95381.

for sulfites in canned and dehydrated fruits and vegetables, jams and jellies, pickles and condiments, fruit juice, frozen potatoes, processed seafood, soup mixes, baked goods, wine, and beer.

❖ **Beware of pesky critters.** If you have dust in your house, you have dust mites. These microscopic creatures leave droppings that cause an allergic reaction in someone with allergies or asthma. Dust mites live everywhere, especially in places at a low altitude or with more than 50 percent humidity. They thrive in carpet, upholstered furniture, mattresses, box springs, pillows, bedcovers, and clothing.

The best way to defeat dust mites is to dust frequently, keep your house as free of clutter as possible, and have lots of smooth surfaces that can be easily cleaned. Vacuum frequently, including mattresses, bedclothes, and curtains. Wear a dust mask when you vacuum to protect yourself. Wash mattress pads, comforters, pillows or pillow covers, and your clothing weekly in hot water. You can also check with your local hardware store to see if they stock acaricide, a substance you can spray on carpets to kill dust mites.

There is some controversy about using foam pillows instead of feather ones. Some studies say foam pillows discourage dust mites, and some say feather pillows do a better job. However, if you enclose mattresses, box springs, and pillows in airtight plastic or allergy-proof covers, that should help keep dust away from you no matter what kind of pillow you choose.

❖ **Be a smoke detector.** Smoke can trigger an asthma attack, whether it comes from a cigarette or a fireplace. Don't let anyone smoke in your home, and avoid places where people are smoking. If you have a fireplace or wood-burning stove in your house, be sure it's vented correctly, and use it as little as possible to avoid aggravating your asthma.

❖ **Take care with furry friends.** Animal dander is a common cause of allergic asthma attacks. If you have a beloved pet that you can't part with, lessen his effect on your asthma by keeping him outside as much as possible. If he must stay inside, give him weekly baths to remove much of the dander that causes problems. (Check with your vet to be sure this won't dry his skin too much.) Keep him out of the bedroom at all costs; your airways are more vulnerable to allergens at night. Have a non-asthmatic family member brush your animal outside and clean his litter box or cage. For a dog, use washable bedding and launder it frequently.

❖ **Halt your heartburn.** If you're bothered by the frequent burning of stomach acid up into your esophagus, you probably have gastroesophageal reflux disease, or GERD for short. This chronic form of indigestion can make your asthma symptoms worse, or even cause them in the first place. If you have GERD, see your doctor to have it treated. You might find your asthma improves as well.

At home, avoid eating or drinking for several hours before you go to bed. Try to eat lightly for your evening meal and see if your nighttime asthma improves. Raising the head of your bed with four-inch blocks may help your GERD as well as your asthma. If your head stays higher than your stomach, you'll keep stomach acid in its place.

❖ **Exercise anyway.** You know exercise is important to your health, but you know it can trigger asthma, too. Be choosy about your exercise, and you can be as active as the next person. Walking, weight training, swimming, baseball, and downhill skiing are your best exercise choices. Be sure to warm up and cool down properly for every exercise session. This gradually increases your strength and lung capacity.

Exercise in clean environments that are warm and humid. Early morning is usually the least polluted time of day in the city. On cold days, wear a scarf or face mask over your nose and mouth to help warm the air. Always breathe through your nose instead of your mouth so the air is warmed and moistened in your nasal passages.

❖ **Be careful of combinations.** The combination of asthma and certain medicines can be dangerous. As many as 20 percent of adults with asthma have attacks from a drug reaction. Watch out for aspirin and other NSAIDS such as ibuprofen and naproxen, beta blockers, antihistamines, ACE inhibitors, and contrast dyes used for X-rays. Double check with your doctor before taking any of these, and let her know immediately if you have problems. Watch yourself carefully for any reaction when you start taking a new medicine.

There are many things you can do to influence the place asthma has in your life. Follow your doctor's orders, be prepared with the medicine you need, and take control of your environment so you can avoid the triggers around you. Along with your actions, keep a hopeful and positive attitude. You should be breathing easier in no time.

Food, vitamin, and mineral chart

	RDA	Foods	Amount
Folic acid	200 mcg	Liver (3.5 oz, fried)	220 mcg
		Avocado (1 medium)	113 mcg
		Spinach (1/2 cup, raw)	54 mcg
		Pinto beans (1 cup, boiled)	294 mcg
		Orange (1 medium)	47 mcg
Iron	10 mg	Ribeye steak (3.5 oz, broiled)	2.34 mg
		Liver (3.5 oz, fried)	6.28 mg
		Lima beans (1 cup, boiled)	4.50 mg
		Tuna (3 oz, canned in water)	2.72 mg
		Chicken (3.5 oz, roasted)	1.21 mg
Niacin	19 mg	Baked potato (with skin)	3.3 mg
		Chicken (3.5 oz, roasted)	8.5 mg
		Ham (3.5 oz, cooked)	5.3 mg
		Rice (1 cup, white enriched)	2.1 mg
		Bagel	1.9 mg
Vitamin C	60 mg	Orange (1 medium)	80 mg
		Cantaloupe (1 cup)	68 mg
		Strawberries (1 cup, raw)	85 mg
		Broccoli (1/2 cup, raw)	41 mg
		Green pepper (1/2 cup raw)	64 mg
Vitamin E	10 mg	Wheat germ oil (1 T)	20.30 mg
		Corn oil (1 T)	1.90 mg
		Mango (1 raw)	2.32 mg
		Peanuts (1 oz)	2.56 mg
		Avocado (1 raw)	2.32 mg
Vitamin K	80 mcg	Broccoli (raw)	132 mcg/100 g
		Spinach (raw)	266 mcg/100 g
		Cauliflower (raw)	191 mcg/100 g
		Turnip greens (raw)	650 mcg/100 g
		Soybean oil	540 mcg/100 g
Zinc	15 mg	Oysters (6 med.)	76.4 mg
		Turkey (dark, 3.5 oz.)	4.16 mg
		Lima beans, cooked (1/2 cup)	2.7 mg
		Wheat germ (2 tbsp.)	1.8 mg
		Yogurt, plain (1 cup)	1.3 mg

Sources

801 Prescription Drugs: Good Effects, Side Effects and Natural Healing Alternatives, FC&A Publishing, Peachtree City, Ga., 1996

A Quick Consumer Guide to Safe Food Handling, Home and Garden Bulletin No. 248, U.S. Department of Agriculture

Abnormalities of Heart Rhythm, A Guide for Parents, American Heart Association National Center, 7272 Greenville Avenue, Dallas, TX 75231-4596

Adverse Reactions to Food Additives, American Academy of Allergy, Asthma and Immunology, Internet WWW address <http://www.aaaai.org/patpub/resource/publicat/tips/tip13.html> retrieved on March 11, 1997

Allergic Contact Dermatitis, American Academy of Allergy, Asthma, and Immunology, Internet WWW address <http://www.aaaai.org/patpub/resource/publicat/tips/tip7.html> retrieved on March 11, 1997

Allergies to Animals, American Academy of Allergy, Asthma and Immunology, Internet WWW address <http://www.aaaai.org/patpub/resource/publicat/tips/tip14.html> retrieved on March 11, 1997

Alternative Medicine, Future Medicine Publishing, Puyallup, Wash., 1993

Alzheimer's Disease — A Scientific Guide for Health Practitioners, Publication No. 84-2251, National Institutes of Health, Bethesda, MD 20892

Alzheimer's Disease, Publication No. 94-3676, National Institutes of Health, Bethesda, MD 20892

American Behavioral Scientist (39,3:249)

American Breath Specialists, Internet WWW address <http://www.breath-care.com/cause.html> retrieved on Feb. 4, 1997

American College of Sports Medicine Fitness Book, Leisure Press, Champaign, Ill., 1992

American Family Physician (47,1:185; 49,1:171; 49,6:1385,1423; 49,7:1617; 50,3:633; 50,8:1701; 51,3:679; 51,5:1151; 52,1:159; 52,5:1347; 52,8:2238; 53,3:891; 53,4:1215,1224,1255; 54,2:438; 54,3:947; 54,4:1253; 54,8:2487; and 55,1:22,141,217)

American Health (XII,8:56)

American Journal of Psychiatry (150,4:3)

Anaphylaxis, American Academy of Allergy, Asthma and Immunology, Internet WWW address <http://www.aaaai.org/patpub/resource/publicat/tips/tip18.html> retrieved on March 11, 1997

Annals of Internal Medicine (16,16:127)

Archives of Family Medicine (5,2:79 and 5,5:259)

Arthritis Today (10,1:10; 10,5:14; and 11,1:37,58)

Arthritis: What Works, St. Martin's Paperback, New York, 1992

Asthma and Allergy Advance (May/June 1996)

Back Works, BookPartners, Seattle, 1993

Be Independent (A Guide for People with Parkinson's Disease), The American Parkinson Disease Association, Inc., 60 Bay St., Suite 401, Staten Island, NY 10301

Before You Call the Doctor, Ballantine Books, New York, 1992

Benign Paroxysmal Positional Vertigo, by Timothy C. Hain, M.D., The Vestibular Disorders Association (VEDA), Internet WWW address <http://www.teleport.com/~veda/bppv.html> retrieved on March 24, 1997

Benign Paroxysmal Positional Vertigo, Otology Online, Internet WWW address <http://www.ears.com/quinn/BENIGN_PAROXYSMAL_VERTIGO.html> retrieved on March 18, 1997

Better Homes & Garden After 40 Health and Medical Guide, Meredith Corporation, Des Moines, Iowa, 1980

Brain Basics: Preventing Strokes, National Institute of Neurological Disorders and Stroke, Internet WWW address <http://www.ninds.nih.gov/healinfo/disorder/stroke/strokehp.htm> retrieved on April 8, 1997

British Journal of Clinical Psychology (34,4:543)

British Medical Journal (310,6971:13; 311,7001:349; 311,7003:489; 311,7012:1055; 312,7031:601; 313,7052:241,253; and 313,7071:1501)

Cardiac Alert (15,3:7)

Care of the Neck, J.B. Lippincott Company, Philadelphia, 1985

Cecil Textbook of Medicine, 19th Edition, W.B. Saunders Co., Philadelphia, 1992

Chest (105,3:968)

Chronic Fatigue Syndrome, Internet WWW address <http://www.niaid.nih.gov/factsheet/cfs.htm> retrieved on June 13, 1997

Compendium of Olfactory Research 1982-1994, Kendall/Hunt Publishing, Dubuque, Iowa, 1995

Complete Guide to Symptoms, Illness & Surgery for People Over 50, The Berkeley Publishing Group, New York, 1992

Complete Guide to Symptoms, Illness & Surgery, The Berkley Publishing Group, New York, 1995

Constipation, National Institute of Diabetes and Digestive and Kidney Diseases, National Institutes of Health, http://www.niddk.nih.gov/Constipation/Constipation.html

Consultant (35,6:803 and 35,11:1621)

Consumer Guide — Family Medical and Health Guide, Publications International, Ltd., Lincolnwood, Ill., 1991

Coping With the Stress of Tinnitus, American Tinnitus Association, P.O. Box 5, Portland, OR 97207-0005

Diabetes in the News (13,6:32)

Diabetes Overview, Publication No. 96-3873, National Institute of Diabetes and Digestive and Kidney Diseases, National Institutes of Health, Bethesda, MD 20892

Diabetes Statistics, Publication No. 96-3926, National Institute of Diabetes and Digestive and Kidney Diseases, National Institutes of Health, Bethesda, MD 20892

Diabetic Neuropathy: The Nerve Damage of Diabetes, Publication No. 95-3185, National Institutes of Health, Bethesda, MD 20892

Diet and Health, National Research Council, National Academy Press, Washington, 1989

Dieting and Gallstones, National Institute of Diabetes and Digestive and Kidney Diseases, National Institutes of Health, Internet WWW address <http://www.niddk.nih.gov/Diet&Gall/Diet&Gall.html> retrieved on July 1, 1997

Digestive Diseases Statistics, National Institute of Diabetes and Digestive and Kidney Diseases, National Institutes of Health, Internet WWW address <http://www.niddk.nih.gov/DD_Statistics/DD_Statistics.html> retrieved on May 22, 1997

Diverticulosis and Diverticulitis, Publication No. 92-1163, National Institute of Diabetes and Digestive and Kidney Diseases, National Institutes of Health, Bethesda, MD 20892

Dr. Dean Ornish's Program for Reversing Heart Disease, Random House, New York, 1990

Drugs and Aging (6,6:465)

Eczema/Atopic Dermatitis, American Academy of Dermatology, Internet WWW address <http://tray.dermatology.uiowa.edu/PIPs/AtopDerm.html> retrieved on Sept. 15, 1996

Emergency Medicine (23,10:20; 28,8:46; and 28,11:64)

Encyclopedia of Natural Medicine, Prima Publishing, Rocklin, Calif., 1991

Encyclopedia of Nutritional Supplements, Prima Publishing, Rocklin, Calif., 1996

Estrogen and Delayed Onset of Alzheimer's Disease, National Institute on Aging News Release (Aug. 16, 1996)

Everything You Need to Know About Diseases, Springhouse Corp., Springhouse, Pa., 1996

Examination of the Link Between Depression and Heart Disease, Internet WWW address <http:www.heartinfo.org/depchd297.htm> retrieved on March 20, 1997

Executive Health Report (25,7:1)

Executive Health's Good Health Report (31,11:1)

Exercise and Your Arthritis, Arthritis Foundation, P.O. Box 19000, Atlanta, GA 30326

Face Pain, Internet WWW address <http://www.familyinternet.com/mhc/top/003027.htm> retrieved on April 1, 1997

Facts About Arrhythmias/Rhythm Disorders, National Heart, Lung, and Blood Institute Communications and Public Information Branch, Building 31, Room 4A21, Bethesda, MD 20892

Facts and Fallacies About Digestive Diseases, Publication No. 95-2673, National Institute of Diabetes and Digestive and Kidney Diseases, National Institutes of Health, Bethesda, MD 20892

Family Medical & Health Guide, Publications International, Ltd., Lincolnwood, Ill., 1991

FDA Consumer (24,10:33; 25,6:36; 26,2:31; 26,7:26; 29,8:14; and 30,7:25)

Fever as Healer, Tom Kruzel, ND, Internet WWW address <http://infinity.dorsai.org/Naturopathic.Physician/articles.lay/ART.fever.tk.html> retrieved on March 8, 1997

Fever Blisters and Canker Sores, American Academy of Otolaryngology — Head and Neck Surgery, Inc., One Prince Street, Alexandria, VA 22314

Fever Blisters and Canker Sores, Publication No. 92-247, National Institute of Dental Research, National Institutes of Health, Bethesda, MD 20892

Fever in Adults, Vancouver Hospital Emergency Medicine, Internet WWW address <http://www.medscene.com/docinhouse/fever_adult.html> retrieved on April 24, 1997

Flu, Office of Communications, National Institute of Allergy and Infectious Diseases, National Institutes of Health, Bethesda, MD 20892

Food and Mood: The Complete Guide to Eating Well and Feeling Your Best, Henry Holt and Co., Inc., New York, 1995

Food Values of Portions Commonly Used, HarperPerennial, New York, 1989

Gallstones, National Institute of Diabetes and Digestive and Kidney Diseases, National Institutes of Health, Internet WWW address <http://www.niddk.nih.gov/Gallstones/Gallstones.html> retrieved on April 30, 1997

Gallstones: A National Health Problem, American Liver Foundation, Cedar Grove, NJ 07009

Gastroesophageal Reflux Disease, Publication No. 94-882, National Institute of Diabetes and Digestive and Kidney Diseases, National Institutes of Health, Bethesda, MD 20892

Geriatrics (50,3:22; 51,4:47; 51,6:18; 51,12:28,45; and 52,2:27)

Griffith's 5 Minute Clinical Consultant, Williams & Wilkins, Baltimore, 1996

Hamilton and Whitney's Nutrition Concepts and Controversies, West Publishing Company, St. Paul, Minn., 1994

Headache — Hope Through Research, Publication No. 84-158, U.S. Department of Health and Human Services, National Institutes of Health, Bethesda, MD 20892

Healing With Food, HarperPerennial, New York, 1993

Health News (2,16:6)

HealthFacts (21,210:1)

Heart and Stroke Facts, American Heart Association National Center, 7272 Greenville Avenue, Dallas, TX 75231-4596

Hemorrhoids, National Institute of Diabetes and Digestive and Kidney Diseases, National Institutes of Health, Internet WWW address <http://www.niddk.gov/hemmorhoids/hemmorhoids.html> retrieved on April 10, 1997

Herbs for Health (1,3:51 and 1,4:34)

Herbs of Choice: The Therapeutic Use of Phytomedicinals, The Haworth Press, Binghamton, N.Y., 1994

High Blood Pressure Lowered Naturally, FC&A Publishing, Peachtree City, Ga., 1995

Holistic Nursing Practice (10,2:49)

Hypoglycemia, Publication No. 95-3926, National Institute of Diabetes and Digestive and Kidney Diseases, National Institutes of Health, Bethesda, MD 20892

Impotence Resource Center, The Geddings Osbon Sr. Foundation, Internet WWW address <http://www.impotence.org/facts.htm> retrieved on March 19, 1997

Impotence, National Institutes of Health Consensus Development Conference Statement, National Institutes of Health, Internet WWW address <http://text.nlm.nih.gov/nih/cdc/www/911txt.html> retrieved on July 3, 1997

Inside the Brain — Revolutionary Discoveries of How the Mind Works,
  Andrews and McMeel, Kansas City, Mo., 1996

Inside Tract, promotional newsletter, Glaxo Wellcome Institute for Digestive
  Health, Research Triangle Park, N.C.

Irritable Bowel Syndrome, National Institute of Diabetes and Digestive and
  Kidney Diseases, National Institutes of Health, WWW address
  <http://www.niddk.nih.gov/IBS/IBS.html> retrieved on Feb. 25, 1997

Ischemic Heart Disease: Angina Pectoris, Scientific American Medicine, New
  York, 1991

Journal of Consulting and Clinical Psychology (63,6:862)

Journal of Family Practice (36:2,207)

Journal of Gerontology, Medical Sciences (52A,1:M27)

Journal of Occupational and Environmental Medicine (38,5:485)

Journal of the American College of Nutrition (15,6:630)

Journal of the American Dietetic Association (95,6:661)

Journal of the American Geriatric Society (44,9:1025)

Lactose Intolerance, Publication No. 94-2751, National Institute of Diabetes
  and Digestive and Kidney Diseases, National Institutes of Health,
  Bethesda, MD 20892

*Life-threatening irregular heart rhythms peak on Monday, Friday — even
  among retired*, American Heart Association News Release (Sept. 15, 1996)

Lifetime Encyclopedia of Natural Remedies, Parker Publishing Co., West
  Nyack, N.Y., 1993

*Lower Educational and Occupational Levels Increase Risk for Alzheimer's
  Disease*, National Institute on Aging News Release (April 5, 1994)

Mayo Clinic Health Letter (11,12:1)

Med Facts: Anaphylaxis, National Jewish Medical and Research Center,
  Internet WWW address <http://www.njc.org/MFhtml/ANA_MF.html>
  retrieved on March 13, 1997

Medical Abstracts Newsletter (13,3:2)

Medical Tribune for the Internist and Cardiologist (36,10:19; 36,13:12; and
  37,10:11)

Mind Over Back Pain, Berkley Books, New York, 1982

Moles, American Academy of Dermatology, Internet WWW address
  <http://tray.dermatology.uiowa.edu/PIPs/Rosacea.html> retrieved on
  Sept. 15, 1996

Nasal Wash Treatment, National Jewish Medical and Research Center,
  Internet WWW address <http://www.njc.org/MFhtml/NSW_MF.html>
  retrieved on April 7, 1997

National Headache Foundation Headlines (86:10 and 94:3)

National Institute of Arthritis and Musculoskeletal and Skin Diseases, 1
  AMS Circle, Bethesda, MD 20892-3675

Natural Medicines and Cures Your Doctor Never Tells You About, FC&A
  Publishing, Peachtree City, Ga., 1995

Natural Prescriptions, Ballantine Books, New York, 1994

Neck Pain, American Academy of Orthopaedic Surgeons, 222 South
  Prospect Avenue, Park Ridge, Ill. 60068

New Study Shows Clothing is an Important Source of Mite Allergen, News
  Release (Jan. 29, 1996), American Academy of Allergy, Asthma and
  Immunology, 611 E. Wells Street, Milwaukee, WI 53202-3889

No More Aching Back, Villard Books, New York, 1990

Noise — Its Effects on Hearing & Tinnitus, American Tinnitus Association, P.O. Box 5, Portland, OR 97207-0005

Nursing (24,5:25)

Nursing 95 Drug Handbook, Springhouse Corp., Springhouse, Pa., 1995

Nutrition Action Health Letter (23,9:1)

Nutrition Research Newsletter (XII,10:103)

Pallidotomy in Brief, Matthias C. Kurth, M.D., Internet WWW address <http://neuro-chief-e.mgh.harvard.edu/parkinsonsweb/Main/Surgery/PDUpdte48.html> retrieved on May 30, 1996

Parkinson's Disease Handbook, The American Parkinson Disease Association, Inc., 60 Bay St., Suite 401, Staten Island, NY 10301

Pharmacy Times (61,3:55 and 62,5:5HPT)

Poison Ivy, Sumac and Oak, American Academy of Dermatology, Internet WWW address <http://tray.dermatology.uiowa.edu/PIPs/PoisonIvy.html> retrieved on Sept. 15, 1996

Popular Antihistamine Linked to Fatal Heart Rhythm Abnormalities, Internet WWW address <http:www.heartinfo.org/seldane297.htm> retrieved on March 20, 1997

Postgraduate Medicine (97,5:206; 99,5:137; 100,2:252; 100,6:107; and 101,1:114)

Present Knowledge in Nutrition, ILSI Press, Washington, 1996

Primary Hyperparathyroidism, Applied Medical Informatics, Inc., Internet WWW address <http://www.familyinternet.com/peds/top/000384.htm> retrieved on March 6, 1997

Professional Nurse (8,8:524)

Psychological Reports (79:83)

Putting Out the Fire of Heartburn, Center for Digestive Health and Nutrition, Internet WWW address <http://www.gihealth.com/Articles/Reflux.html> retrieved on June 26, 1997

Recognizing Asthma Signs and Symptoms, National Jewish Medical and Research Center, Internet WWW address <http://www.njc.org/MFhtml/Ras_MF.html> retrieved on March 13, 1997

Removing House Dust and Other Allergic Irritants from Your Home, American Academy of Allergy, Asthma and Immunology, Internet WWW address<http://www.aaaai.org/patpub/resource/publicat/tips/tip2.html> retrieved on March 11, 1997

Research may help workers avoid carpal tunnel syndrome, Purdue University News Release (February 1997)

Rosacea Review (Spring 1996, Fall 1996)

Rosacea Tripwires, National Rosacea Society, 800 S. Northwest Hwy., Suite 200, Barrington, IL 60010

Rosacea, Internet WWW address <http://tray.dermatology.uiowa.edu/PIPs/Rosacea.html> retrieved on June 10, 1997

Rosacea, What You Should Know, Galderma Laboratories, Inc, P.O. Box 331329, Fort Worth, TX 76163

Science News (150,25-26:388)

SHHH Journal (17,1:16)

Sinusitis, National Jewish Medical and Research Center, Internet WWW address <http://njc.org/MFhtml/SIN_MF.html> retrieved on April 7, 1997

Sleep Apnea, Internet WWW address <http://www.aomc.org/NR_sleepap-nea.html> retrieved on March 14, 1997

Sleep Apnea, Internet WWW address <http://www.njc.org/PRhtml/!k_Apnea.htm> retrieved on March 14, 1997

Social Science and Medicine (38,8:1037)

Stomach and Duodenal Ulcers, Publication No. 95-38, National Institute of Diabetes and Digestive and Kidney Diseases, National Institutes of Health, Bethesda, MD 20892

Super Healing Foods, Parker Publishing Company, West Nyack, N.Y., 1995

Surgical Neurology (39:5)

Symptoms, Bantam Books, New York, 1989

Symptoms, Illness & Surgery, The Berkley Publishing Group, New York, 1995

Systemic Lupus Erythematosus, Internet WWW address <http://www.njc.org/MPhtml/SLE_MP.html> retrieved on March 25, 1997

Take Care of Yourself, Addison-Wesley Publishing Co., New York, 1996

Taking Care of Your Foot and Ankle, American Physical Therapy Association, 1996

The American Journal of Clinical Nutrition (62,6:1212)

The American Journal of Sports Medicine (23,2:251)

The American Medical Association Complete Guide to Women's Health, Random House, New York, 1996

The American Medical Association Encyclopedia of Medicine, Random House, New York, 1989

The American Medical Association Family Medical Guide, Random House, New York, 1994

The American Medical Association Guide to Your Family's Symptoms, Random House, New York, 1992

The Atlanta Journal/Constitution (May 3, 1994, E5; Dec. 12, 1996, C2; Jan. 31, 1997, F-2; March 13, 1997, E3; March 19, 1997, D3; March 20, 1997, B3; and April 2, 1997, B3)

The Big Book of Health Tips, FC&A Publishing, Peachtree City, Ga., 1996

The CFIDS Chronicle (1,1:14 and 9,4:46)

The Columbia University College of Physicians and Surgeons Complete Medical Guide, Crown Publishers, Inc., New York, 1995

The Complete Life Encyclopedia, Thomas Nelson Publishers, Nashville, Tenn., 1990

The Diabetes Advisor (5,1:14)

The Doctor's Complete Guide to Vitamins and Minerals, Bantam Doubleday Dell Publishing Group, New York, 1994

The Essential Guide to Vitamins and Minerals, HarperPerennial, New York, 1995

The Fit or Fat Target Diet, Houghton Mifflin Company, Boston, 1984

The Home Remedies Handbook, Publications International, Ltd., Lincolnwood, Ill., 1993

The Honest Herbal, Varro E. Tyler, Ph.D., The Haworth Press, Binghamton, N.Y., 1993

The Johns Hopkins White Papers, The Johns Hopkins Medical Institutions, Baltimore, 1997

The Journal of Nutrition (125,3S:639,733)

The Journal of the American Medical Association (265,22:3014; 269,14:1836; 272,19:1489; 273,5:402; 275,21:1672; 276,20:1631; and 277,1:25)

The Lancet (345,8944:229; 347,9000:494; 347,9001:604; 347,9009:1159; 347,9014:1507; and 348,9040:1467)

The New England Journal of Medicine (331,2:69; 332,6:351; 333,10:609; and 333,14:913)

The New York Times (Dec. 14, 1989)

The Newnan Times-Herald (Feb. 14, 1996, 4B)

The Physician and Sportsmedicine (22,7:66; 22,11:87; 23,7:79; and 24,2:33)

The Secret of Good Posture, American Physical Therapy Association, 111 North Fairfax Street, Alexandria, VA 22314

Tips on Good Foot Care, National Institute of Diabetes and Digestive and Kidney Diseases, National Institutes of Health, Internet WWW address <http://www.niddk.nih.gov/FootCare/Tips.html> retrieved on April 29, 1997

To Sleep..., Atlanta Center for Sleep Disorders at Georgia Baptist Medical Center, 300 Boulevard NE, Box 44, Atlanta, GA 30312

Tracking and treating lupus — the great imposter, Brian L. Kotzin, M.D., Internet WWW address <http:/www.njc.org/MSU/09n4MSU_Lupus.html> retrieved on April 4, 1997

Triggers of Asthma, American Academy of Allergy, Asthma and Immunology, Internet WWW address <http://www.aaaai.org/patpub/resource/ publicat/tips/tip4.html> retrieved on March 11, 1997

Tufts University Diet & Nutrition Letter (14,10:1)

U.S. Pharmacist (17,6:17; 21,11:12; and 22,1:22)

Understanding Angina, American Heart Association, 7272 Greenville Ave., Dallas, TX 75231–4596

Understanding the Pollen and Mold Season, American Academy of Allergy, Asthma and Immunology, Internet WWW address <http://www.aaaai.org/patpub/resource/publicat/tips/tip8.html> retrieved on March 11, 1997

Urinary Tract Infections in Adults, Publication No. 91-2097, National Institute of Diabetes and Digestive and Kidney Diseases, National Institutes of Health, Bethesda, MD 20892

Using Your Joints Wisely, Arthritis Foundation, P.O. Box 19000, Atlanta, GA 30326

Varicose Veins and Haemorrhoids: Prevention and Treatment, Leon Chaitow, Internet WWW address <http://www.healthy.net/library/ articles/Chaitow/VARICOSE.HTM> retrieved on March 26, 1997

Varicose Veins, American Institute of Preventive Medicine, Internet WWW address <http://205.180.229.2/library/books/healthyself/womens/ vveins.htm> retrieved on March 26, 1997

Varicose Veins, David L. Hoffman, Internet WWW address <http://www.healthy.net/library/Hoffman/Cardiovascular/varicose.htm> retrieved on March 26, 1997

Varicose Veins, Internet WWW address <http://web.bu.edu/COHIS/ cardvasc/vessel/vein/varicose.html> retrieved on March 26, 1997

What Is An Allergic Reaction? American Academy of Allergy, Asthma and Immunology, Internet WWW address, <http://www.aaaai.org/patpub/ resource/publicat/tips/tip5.html> retrieved on March 11, 1997

What is Non-Insulin-Dependent Diabetes? American Diabetes Association, Diabetes Information Service Center, 1660 Duke Street, Alexandria, VA 22314

What is Sjogren's Syndrome? National Sjogren's Syndrome Association, Internet WWW address <http://www.sjogrens.org/what.htm> retrieved on May 13, 1997

What You Need to Know About Diabetes, American Diabetes Association, Diabetes Information Service Center, 1660 Duke Street, Alexandria, VA 22314

What You Need to Know About Periodontal (Gum) Diseases, National Institute of Dental Research, P.O. Box 54793, Washington, DC 20032

Women's Health Companion, Celestial Arts, Berkeley, Calif., 1995

Worst Pills Best Pills II, Public Citizen's Research Group, 1993

Index